TRAUMATIC DISLOCATION
OF THE HIP

TRAUMATIC DISLOCATION OF THE HIP

Herman C. Epstein, M.D.

Clinical Professor Emeritus
Department of Orthopaedic Surgery
University of Southern California
Los Angeles, California

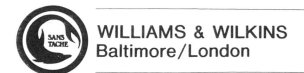

WILLIAMS & WILKINS
Baltimore/London

LONQML J

Library of Congress Cataloging in Publication Data

Epstein, Herman C
    Traumatic dislocation of the hip.

    Bibliography: p.
    Includes index.
    1. Hip joint—Dislocation. 2. Hip joint—Wounds and injuries. 3. Hip joint—Surgery. I. Title.
RD549.E67   617'.16   79-9482
ISBN 0-683-02906-1

Composed and printed at the
Waverly Press, Inc.
Mt. Royal and Guilford Aves.
Baltimore, Md. 21202, U.S.A.

This monograph is dedicated to my teachers, to my friend, the late Vernon Thompson, M.D., and to my wife Beatrice, who has stood by me through all these years.

FOREWORD

This monograph represents the current thoughts of a man who has thought about this problem for more than 30 years. Although this man is retired, I would not wish to feel that this is a culmination of efforts nor an end point. It is merely another step in a long-term study and dedication to an interesting orthopaedic problem on the part of Dr. Herman Epstein.

Any good scientific study may answer to some degree a question, but if it is a good study, it opens a host of new problems which deserve even more work and opens up new vistas and paths in the quest for knowledge.

The original study was started in the mid-1940's and the preliminary report was given at the Western Orthopaedic Association meeting in 1949. The following year, with probability figures added for the first time in the orthopaedic literature, the first paper was presented at the annual meeting of the American Academy of Orthopaedic Surgeons. It was awarded the Kappa Delta Award on the basis of using the probability figures in such a statistical analysis.

The natural outcome of this presentation was to study the method of treatment and perhaps devise a method to provide better results than found in this study. Thus, nine more years of study and effort produced a paper presented at the annual meeting of the American Academy of Orthopaedic Surgeons in 1958 comparing open and closed method of treatment of posterior fracture-dislocation of the hip with some definite recommendations and again some obvious questions unanswered.

This study continues. Dr. Epstein has provided transportation at his own expense for patients to return for follow-up studies. He has advised and helped in the management of hip dislocations in this large county hospital over all these years. He continues to read and think about the problem. He has attempted to stimulate others to carry on the clinical studies and to study the effects of damages on cartilage and bone.

We all appreciate and applaud this effort. Those of us close to Dr. Epstein realize it is but one more step in an unending path pursued by a man who was stimulated by a fine orthopaedic surgeon, Dr. V. P. Thompson initially, who is presently carrying the burden almost alone and who is continuously stimulating others to pick up this problem and carry it further.

J. Paul Harvey, Jr., M.D.
Chief Physician
Department of Orthopedic Surgery
Los Angeles County-University of Southern California Medical Center

ACKNOWLEDGMENTS

The following are some names of people who have been directly concerned with my studies on traumatic dislocations of the hip and those who have been helpful in making this monograph possible.

I am most grateful to the late Drs. Donald Blanche and Harold Crowe, who encouraged me to continue with my studies, first as an orthopaedic resident and later as a practicing orthopaedist. Dr. J. Paul Harvey, Jr., Chief Physician of the Orthopedic Department, Los Angeles County-University of Southern California Medical Center, has been very helpful in arranging that I saw all traumatic dislocated hips either at the time of injury or at the trauma clinic. His associate professors, Drs. Michael Patzakis and Tillman Moore, have also contributed greatly. Dr. Augusto Sarmiento, Lowman Professor and Chairman, USC Department of Orthopedics, has read the text and made suggestions.

I wish to thank the following doctors who have contributed cases: Harvard Ellman, my former associate in practice; Lester Cohn and Howard Hirsch, Chief Orthopedists at the Veterans Hospital in Sepulveda; William Stryker, J. Harold LaBriola, John Rieder, and Chad Smith at the Orthopedic Hospital; Saul Bernstein, John King, and John C. Wilson at the Childrens Hospital; and John D. Hsu and Vernon Nickel at Rancho Los Amigos Hospital. Other doctors who contributed are Robert Nippell, Homer Graham, Fred Polesky, George Wiesseman, Charles Owen, Alonzo Neufeld, Ian Brodie, Frank Schiller, Stanford Noel, Klaus Odenheimer, Richard Saxon, and Vernon Luck.

I want to especially thank Dr. Brent for his help with type I dislocations. Also thanks to Dr. Bernard Kahn for his photographs taken of an anterior pubic dislocation.

I am grateful for x-ray films given me by the Kodak Company when follow-up cases were examined at my office. For the beautiful drawings made by Benita Epstein, thanks. The excellent photographs are the work of Lloyd Matlovsky and Andy Gero from the Los Angeles County Hospital, and Susan Sparling, Orthopedic Hospital.

The statistical analysis of the data presented was through the efforts of John M. Weiner, Ph.D., Department of Medicine, University of Southern California. This monograph would have been impossible without the help of Pecolia Murphy, who was in charge of obtaining the records and roentgenograms. And to Dorothy Preston, Carol Marquez and Ruth Kadish, thanks are due for their help in typing this manuscript. And last but not least, to all the orthopaedic residents over the many years at the University of Southern California-Los Angeles County Medical Center, who were able to recognize a dislocated hip and notify me as to closed or open procedures.

CONTENTS

CHAPTER
1

INTRODUCTION

Traumatic dislocations of the hip, once considered an infrequent injury, have become more of a problem in the past 10 years. Still it is difficult for any one observer to accumulate a series large enough for a proper statistical study of this important injury. Wearing seatbelts in automobiles could eliminate most of these serious hip injuries since at least 70% of traumatic dislocations were due to automobile accidents. The great increase in all types of motor vehicle accidents and failure to use seat belts have contributed to this increase in traumatic dislocations of the hip.

Thompson and I[100] reported on a survey of 204 cases of traumatic dislocations of the hip in February 1950, covering a period of 21 years from July 1928 to July 1949 (average, 10 dislocations per year).

Because of my continued interest in this serious injury, a total of 830 dislocations have been analyzed. In this 48-year period, from July 1928 to July 1976, the average number of traumatic dislocations of the hip had increased to 24 per year. Although not used in the statistics, at least ten new dislocated hips were treated per month at the Los Angeles County-University of Southern California (LAC-USC) Medical Center during the past 2 years.

The majority of patients were treated at the LAC-USC Medical Center. Some were seen at the Orthopaedic Hospital and the Children's Hospital in Los Angeles and at the Veteran's Hospital, Sepulveda, California, and a small group were treated by me privately.

I examined most of the patients with dislocations at the time of injury or at follow-up or at both times. The remainder were seen by other orthopaedists associated with the Medical Center. No questionnaire evaluations were used. Although many patients had been lost to follow-up at the Medical Center, they were traced and then examined in my office.

The prompt recognition of the dislocation and treatment of most of the patients, considering the high incidence of serious associated injuries, must be credited to the resident staff.

The chief fault in the material is the lack of repeated observations, especially in those cases with a longer follow-up period. Standards for the selection of cases and for methods of evaluation were, therefore, carefully considered in order to make up for this defect as far as possible.

In the study to be discussed there were 830 anterior and posterior dislocations and fracture-dislocations of the hip (Table 1.1).

Sixty-seven percent were between 16 and 40 years of age (Table 1.2). Nine percent were between 2 and 15 years of age. Twenty-five percent of all dislocations occurred in females. Eleven percent of the dislocations were of the anterior type. Eighteen deaths occurred within 1 to 10 days because of severe multiple injuries (Tables 1.3 and 1.4). There were nine bilateral dislocations, one bilateral anterior, one bilateral posterior and seven with an anterior dislocation on one side and a posterior dislocation on the other.

Table 1.1
Distribution of 830 Traumatic Dislocations of the Hip by Type and Sex

	Number of dislocations	Percentage of dislocations
Type of dislocation		
Anterior	93	11
Posterior	737	89
Total	830	100
Sex		
Male	620	75
Female	210	25
Total	830	100

3

Table 1.2
Distribution of 830 Traumatic Dislocations of the Hip by Age Group[a]

Age in years	Number of dislocations	Percentage of series
0–15	75	9.0
16–30	368	45.0
31–40	181	22.0
41–50	109	13.0
51–60	61	7.0
61–80	36	4.0
Total	830	100.0

[a] Ages 16–40 comprise 67% of series; age range, 2–79 years.

Table 1.3
Total Number of Traumatic Dislocations of the Hip According to Type[a]

Type	Sufficient follow-up	Insufficient follow-up	Grand total	Percent of dislocations
I	134	142	276	34
II	43	19	62	7
III	134	40	174	21
IV	69	8	77	9
V	46	9	55	7
Children	51	24	75	9
Anterior	54	39	93	11
Died		18	18	2
Total	531	299	830	100

[a] Adequate follow-up in 64.0% of dislocations. Nine patients had bilateral dislocations.

Table 1.4
Total Number of Traumatic Dislocations of the Hip[a]

Type	Sufficient follow-up	Insufficient follow-up	Grand total
I	134	142	276
II	43	19	62
III	134	40	174
IV	69	8	77
V	46	9	55
Children	51	24	75
Anterior	54	39	93
Died		18	18
Total	531	299	830

[a] Percentage with adequate follow-up, 64.0%; nine with bilateral dislocations.

MATERIALS AND METHODS

Of the 830 dislocations, 299 were excluded from this study for either one of two reasons. First, because the result could not be properly ascertained. For instance, no patients not physically or roentgenographically examined was included on negative evidence alone. (Fifteen patients readmitted to the hospital for other conditions were not included because there was no mention of the hip in the new history, no note made in the physical examination, and no follow-up roentgenogram of the hip. Two former patients, treated as children, reported by telephone, 10 and 13 years after injury, respectively, that they had no symptoms but there was no other confirmation and they were not included in the series.) Second, patients with a good result were not included if they had been followed for less than 1 year. However, since only three patients had an initial fair result which later improved enough to be classified as good, it was decided to include all cases classified as having a fair or poor result, even if the period of follow-up was less than 1 year.

Of the total of 262 patients with fair or poor results, 69 had a follow-up of less than 1 year. Exclusion of these 299 dislocations leaves a series of 531 cases considered suitable for analysis.

One hundred and eighty-five cases (35%) were followed for 5 to 27 years, and 75 (14%) for over 10 years. The average periods of follow-up were as follows: children 78.6 months; anterior dislocations, 70.4 months; type I posterior dislocations, 77.8 months; and posterior fracture dislocations, 71.15 months. The overall average was 74.5 months (Table 1.5).

Table 1.5
Average Follow-up, in Months, in 531 Dislocated Hips with Sufficient Follow-up

Type	Average follow-up (months)	Total number of dislocations
I	77.8	134
II	68.2	43
III	72.4	134
IV	68.4	69
V	66.6	46
Children	78.6	51
Anterior	70.4	54
Total (average)	74.34	531

Table 1.6
Mechanism of Injury

Mechanism	Children	Anterior	Type I	Type II	Type III	Type IV	Type V	Died	Total	Percent
Auto accident	25	54	183	58	141	69	44	13	586	71.0
Auto turned over	0	0	2	2	4	0	1		9	
Motorcycle accident	5	10	37	2	28	5	5	2	84	
Thrown from auto			1						1	
Pedestrian vs. auto	11	10	19	0	2	1	3	3	49	
Bicycle accident	2	0	1	0	1	0	0		4	
Miscellaneous (falls, stairs, etc.)	22	13	17	0	2	1	2		57	
Airplane accident					1				1	
Football	5	0	7	0	1				13	
Volleyball sliding accident			2						2	
Collapse of building	2	1	0	0	1				4	
Fall from second story			2						2	
Fall from horse	1	0	0	0	1				2	
Battered child	1								1	
Heavy object fell on child	1								1	
Auto rear-ended						2			2	
Wrestling		1							1	
Beaten up		2	3						5	
Overturned		1							1	
Aboard ship—struck by object		1							1	
Stepped in hole			1			1			2	
Fell off ladder			1						1	
Total	75	93	276	62	174	77	55	19	830	

The majority of dislocations in this series occurred in automobile accidents when a knee struck the dashboard, forcing the head of the femur out posteriorly if the knee was held in internal rotation and the hip flexed upon impact. If the thigh was abducted, impact upon the knee would cause further abduction and external rotation of the hip, leading to an anterior dislocation. In a few instances impact at the time of collision caused the vehicle's motor to loosen and forced the foot backward with the knee extended, leading to a posterior dislocation. Overturning of a vehicle or ejection of a passenger from a motor vehicle were also causes of both anterior and posterior dislocations of the hip. These results may be attributed directly to failure to use seatbelts although in one known case the seat belt was used but was not fastened tightly. Other causes of traumatic dislocations were auto vs. pedestrian, motorcycle accidents, miscellaneous falls (From bed, down stairs, tripping, etc.), and sports including football, volleyball, skiing, and one baseball accident not used in the statistics. (Table 1.6 and Figs. 1.1–1.13).

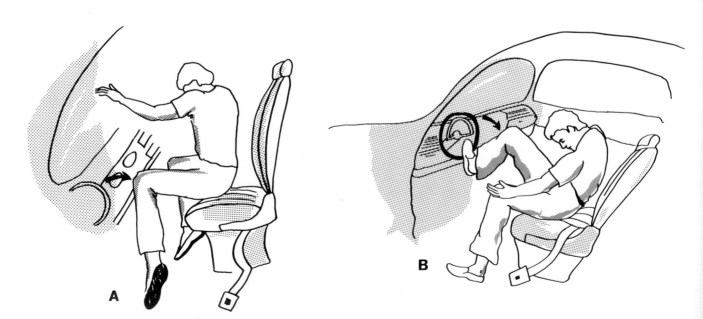

Fig. 1.1 *A* and *B*, the most common cause of posterior dislocations of the hip is the dashboard injury. With the rapid deceleration, the knee strikes against the dashboard and with the hip flexed and adducted, the tremendous thrust on the knee forces the hip out posteriorly. Would wearing a seatbelt properly have prevented this serious injury?

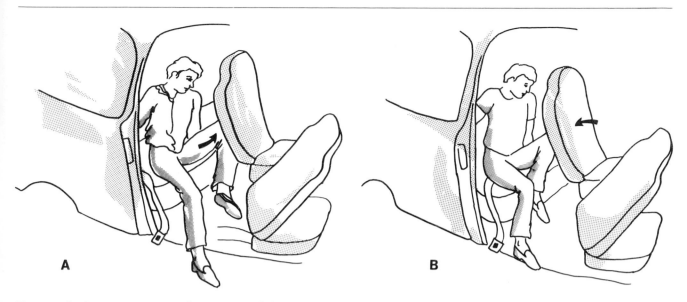

Fig. 1.2 *A,* this patient sustained an *anterior dislocation* of his left hip while sitting in the back seat of an automobile with the lower extremity abducted, in an auto vs. auto collision. Wearing a seatbelt may have prevented the forward thrust of the knee against the front seat of the car. *B,* passengers in the back seat of automobiles may sustain posterior dislocations as occurred in this 15-year-old male.

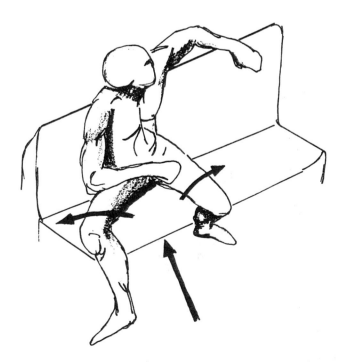

Fig. 1.3 Mechanism of injury of bilateral dislocated hips with wide abduction. Impact of knees against dashboard dislocated both hips.

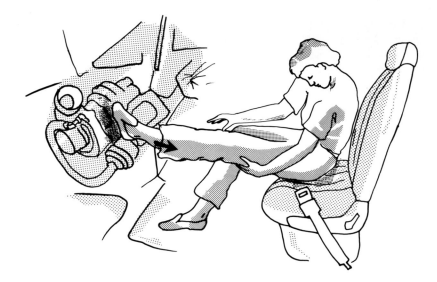

Fig. 1.4 A posterior dislocation may be caused, as in this case, by impact of the dislodged engine striking against the foot with the knee extended. This was the mechanism of injury in three cases.

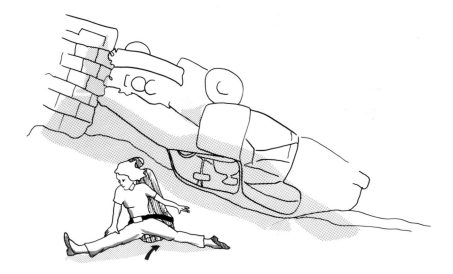

Fig. 1.5 Mechanism of injury causing an obturator dislocation of the left hip. Although the patient was wearing a seatbelt, the impact caused the seat and the patient along with the seatbelt to be thrown out of the automobile.

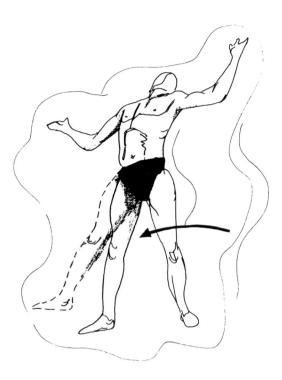

Fig. 1.6 Mechanism of dislocation in patient swimming in ocean and overturned by wave. This caused an anterior pubic dislocation with fracture of the acetabulum.

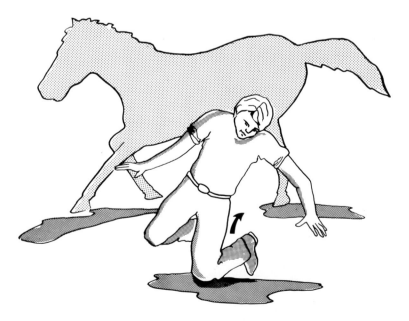

Fig. 1.7 A posterior dislocation occurred when this 10-year-old male fell off a horse, striking his left knee.

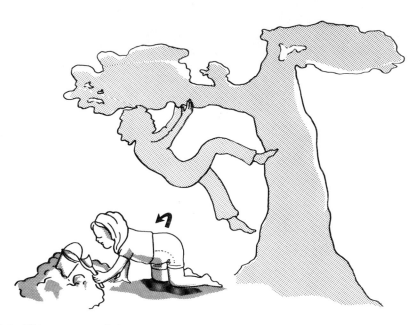

Fig. 1.8 This posterior dislocation occurred in this child when her sister fell out of a tree, landing on the child's back while she was crawling on her hands and knees.

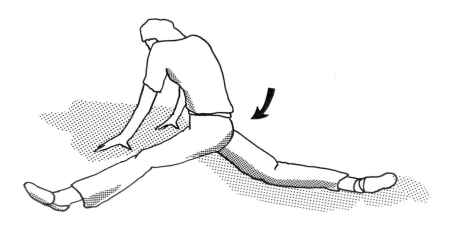

Fig. 1.9 Anterior dislocations, especially in children, may be caused by "trivial injuries." This 6-year-old male slipped and fell with his right hip abducted.

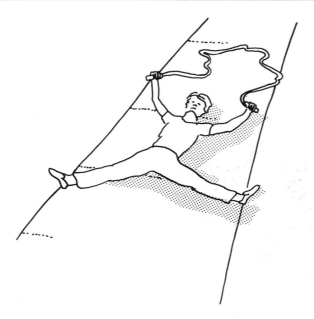

Fig. 1.10 This child was playing and fell backward with wide abduction of his left hip, thus causing an obturator dislocation.

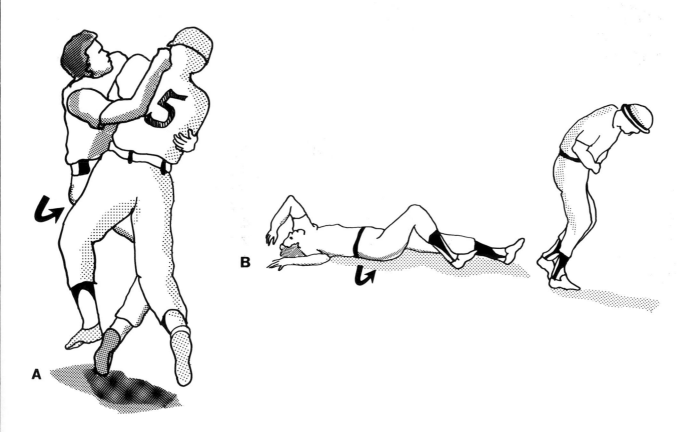

Fig. 1.11 A and B, this posterior dislocation occurred during a collision in a baseball game. This picture was taken from the *Los Angeles Times* and the dislocation was confirmed by the team physician. This case is not used in the statistics.

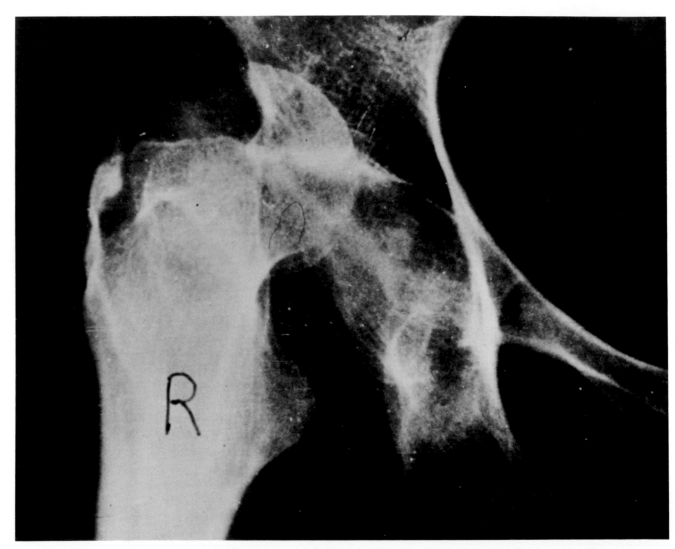

Fig. 1.12   A pubic dislocation without fracture.

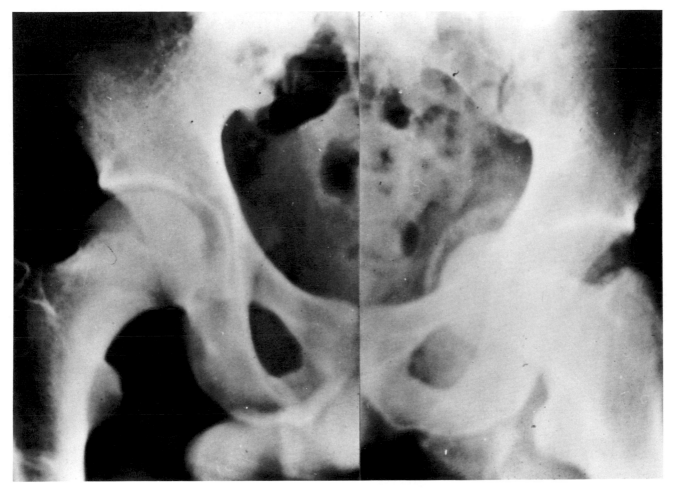

Fig. 1.13 A pubic anterior dislocation 3½ weeks after injury. The femoral head lies anterior to the superior pubic ramus. Note the new bone formation surrounding the femoral head.

CLASSIFICATION OF INJURY

Dislocations were divided into anterior and posterior groups. The anterior dislocations were subdivided into public and obturator with and without fractures. (Table 1.7 and Figs. 1.14–1.22).

There have been many different methods of classifying posterior dislocations and fracture-dislocations.[3, 9, 12, 55, 62, 89, 95] The Thompson and Epstein[100] classification of posterior dislocations is used in this study. The five types of posterior dislocations (Figs. 1.23–1.27) are:

Type I: With or without minor fracture.

Type II: With a large single fracture of the posterior acetabular rim.

Type III: With a comminuted fracture of the rim of the acetabulum, with or without a major fragment.

Table 1.7
Anterior Dislocations

A. Pubic (superior)	B. Obturator (inferior)
With no fracture (simple)	With no fracture (simple)
With fracture, head of femur	With fracture, head of femur
With fracture, acetabulum	With fracture, acetabulum

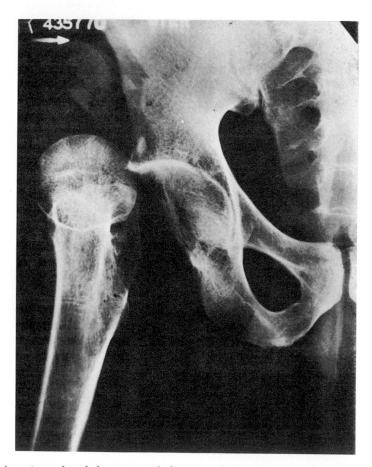

Fig. 1.14 Anterior pubic dislocation with fracture of ilium. (From Epstein, H. C.: Traumatic anterior and simple posterior dislocations of the hip in adults and chidren. In *The American Academy of Orthopaedic Surgeons: Instructional Course Lectures*, vol. 22. The C. V. Mosby Co., St. Louis, 1973. Reproduced with permission.)

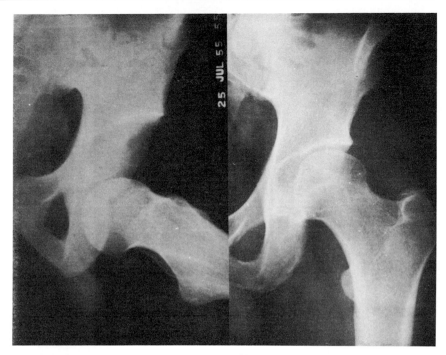

Fig. 1.15 A simple anterior obturator dislocation before and after a closed reduction.

Type IV: With fracture of the acetabular rim and floor.

Type V: With fracture of the femoral head. This classification divides the dislocations with acetabular rim fractures into two groups and excluded central protrusion fractures without posterior dislocation.

After reduction many of the type IV cases had the appearance of central fractures with medial displacement of the head. The extent and comminution of the accompanying fractures occasionally make precise classification difficult. However, for purposes of this study, the classification has been satisfactory.

The attitude of a dislocation is important in determining whether it is anterior or posterior. (Figs. 1.28–1.31).

At times it may be difficult to demonstrate whether a hip is dislocated or whether reduction has been accomplished. If the lesser trochanter is not visualized on anteroposterior views after an attempt at reduction, there is a possibility that the dislocation has not been reduced (Fig. 1.32A–C). Internal and external obliques of the pelvis may be necessary, especially for comminuted fractures of the acetabulum. (Fig. 1.33). A lateral view is important both for anterior and posterior dislocations. (Figs. 1.34 and 1.35). Pain is a definite factor in positioning a patient, so that if oblique views are impractical, stereo roentgenograms would be useful.

In this series there were 61 anterior dislocations (54 in adults and seven in children), 172 posterior type I dislocations (134 in adults, 38 in children), 43 posterior type II dislocations (all in adults), 137 posterior type III dislocations (134 in adults, three in children), 71 posterior type IV dislocations (69 in adults and two in children), and 47 type V posterior dislocations (46 in adults and one in a child). Among the type V cases there were six with an associated fracture of the femoral neck and seven in which the posterior acetabular rim, as well as the femoral head, was fractured.

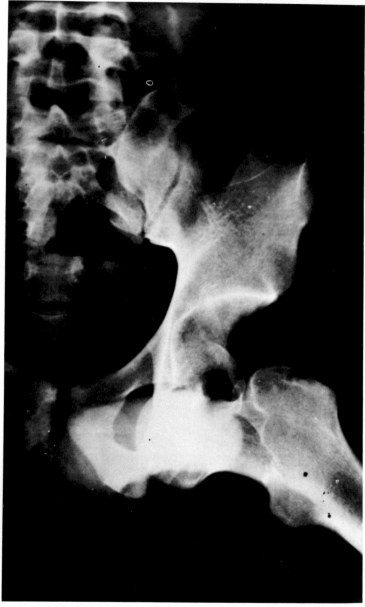

Fig. 1.16 Anterior dislocation with fracture of the femoral head. (From Epstein, H. C.: Traumatic anterior and simple posterior dislocations of the hip in adults and chidren. In *The American Academy of Orthopaedic Surgeons: Instructional Course Lectures,* vol. 22. The C. V. Mosby Co., St. Louis, 1973. Reproduced with permission.)

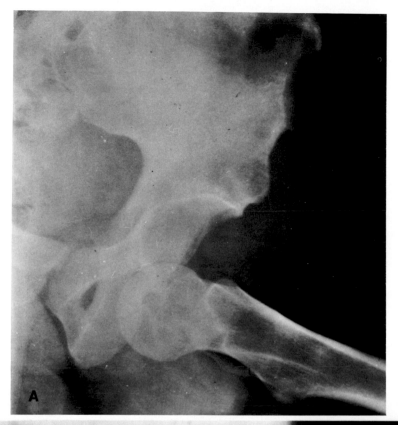

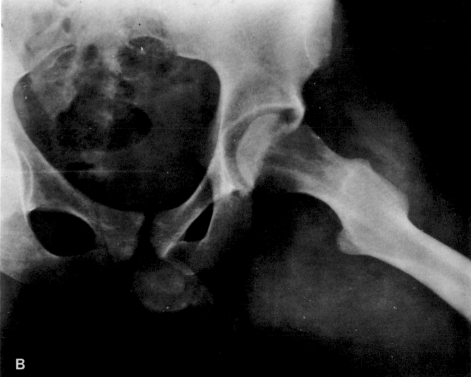

Fig. 1.17 *A,* roentgenogram of obturator dislocation, anterior-posterior view. The femoral head appears normal. *B,* lateral view reveals compression of the femoral head.

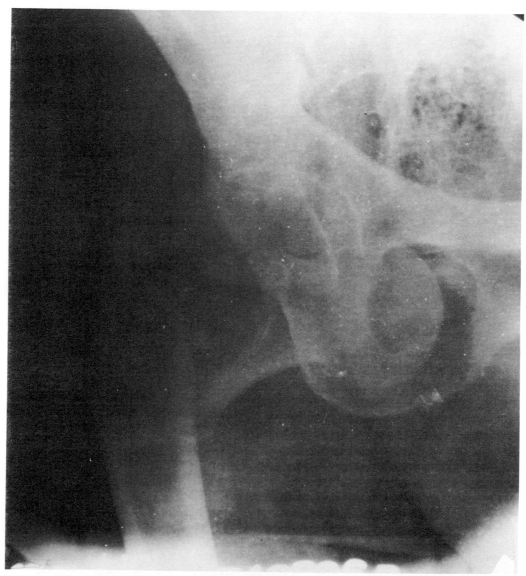

Fig. 1.18   Anterior obturator dislocation with fracture of greater trochanter.

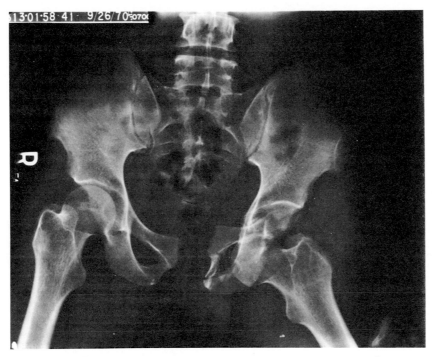

Fig. 1.19 Anterior obturator dislocation left hip with fracture of superior pubic ramus.

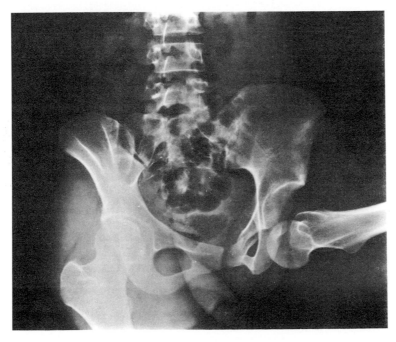

Fig. 1.20 An anterior dislocation with a fracture of the pubic bone.

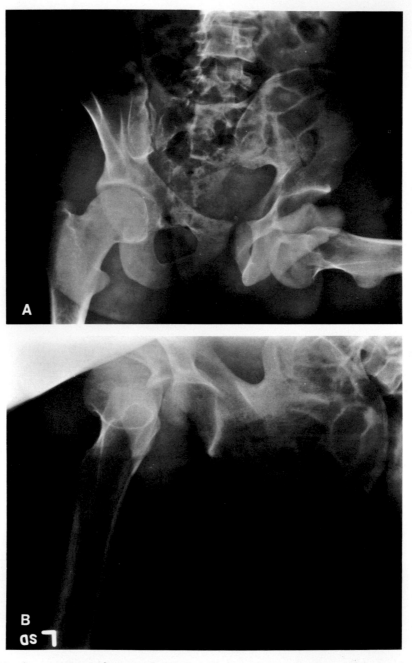

Fig. 1.21 *A,* an anterior obturator dislocation. *B,* lateral view; the femoral head is displaced anteriorly above the acetabulum.

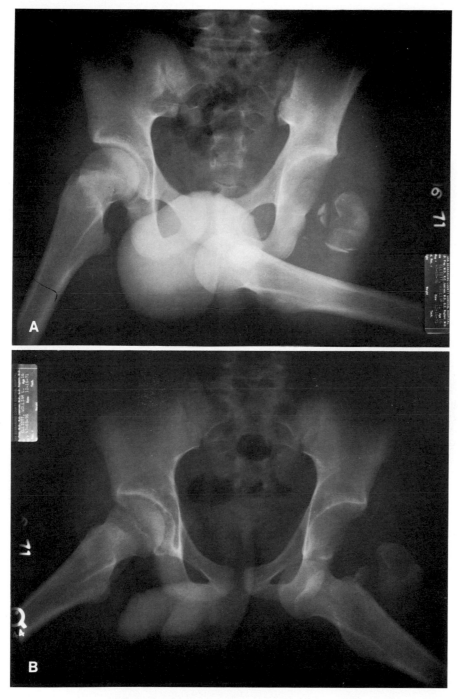

Fig. 1.22 *A* and *B,* an obturator dislocation displaced into the scrotal area. Note the avulsion of the greater trochanter.

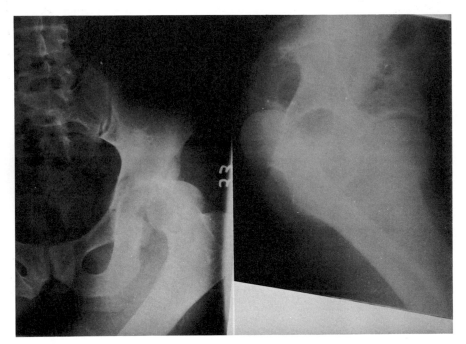

Fig. 1.23   Anterior-posterior and lateral view of posterior dislocation of the hip.

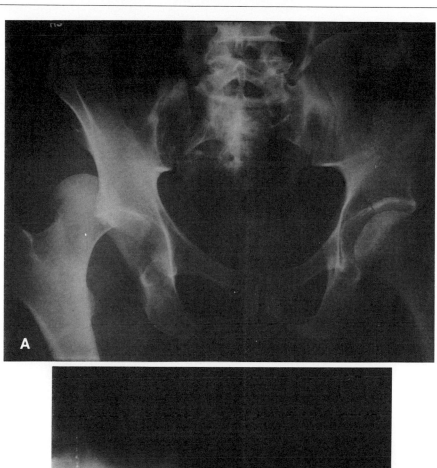

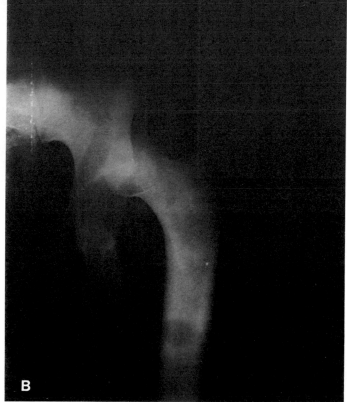

Fig. 1.24 *A* and *B*, type I posterior dislocation without fracture.

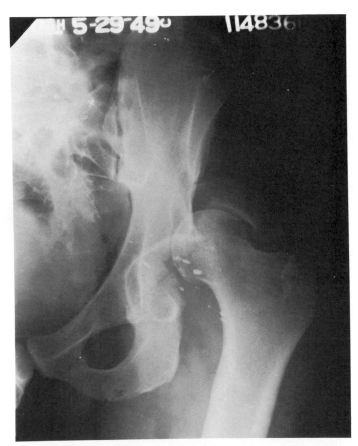

Fig. 1.25   Type II posterior dislocation with large fracture of the posterior acetabular rim.

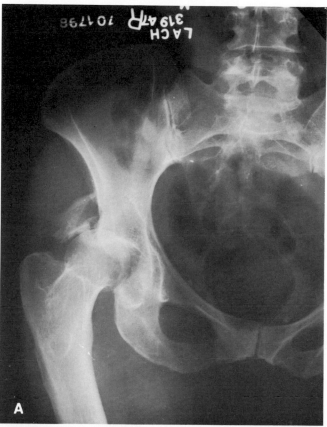

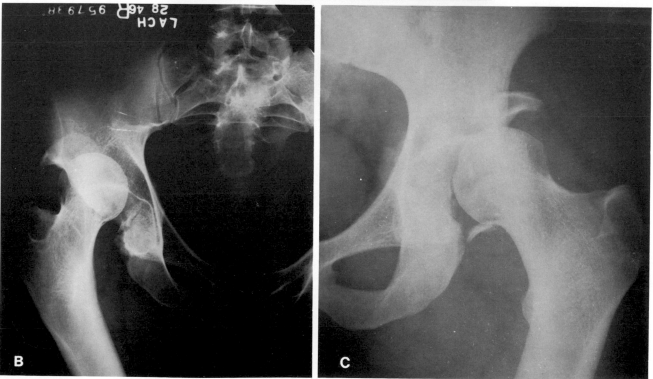

Fig. 1.26 *A, B,* and *C,* three views of a type III classification posterior dislocation with comminuted fracture of rim of acetabulum with or without a major fragment.

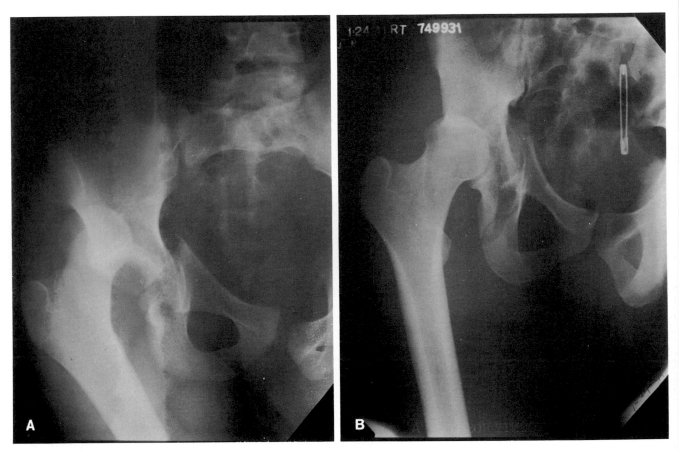

Fig. 1.27   *A,* type IV posterior dislocation through triradiate cartilage. *B,* type IV posterior dislocation with fracture of the acetabular rim and floor.

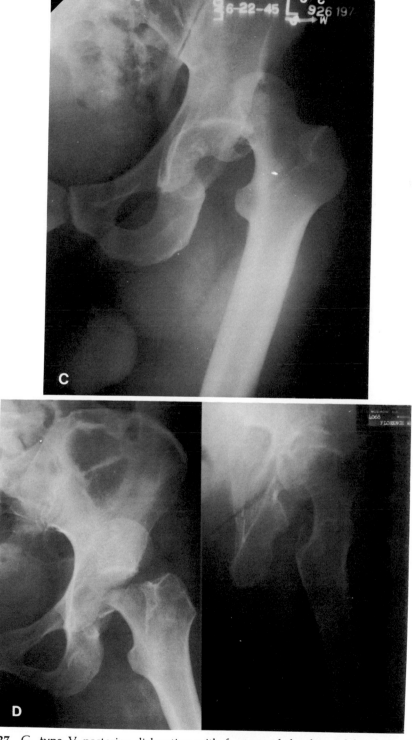

Fig. 1.27 *C,* type V posterior dislocation with fracture of the femoral head. *D,* type V dislocation with a fracture of femoral head and neck of femur.

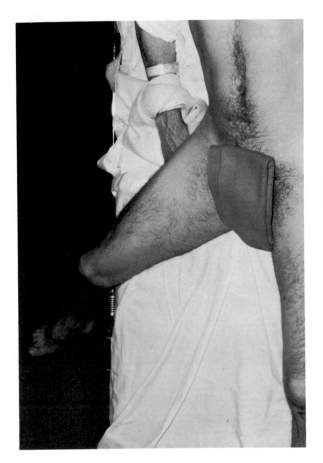

Fig. 1.28 Attitude of an anterior dislocation of right hip. Note abduction, flexion, and external rotation of the hip.

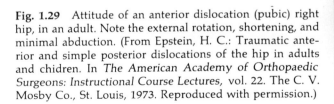

Fig. 1.29 Attitude of an anterior dislocation (pubic) right hip, in an adult. Note the external rotation, shortening, and minimal abduction. (From Epstein, H. C.: Traumatic anterior and simple posterior dislocations of the hip in adults and chidren. In *The American Academy of Orthopaedic Surgeons: Instructional Course Lectures,* vol. 22. The C. V. Mosby Co., St. Louis, 1973. Reproduced with permission.)

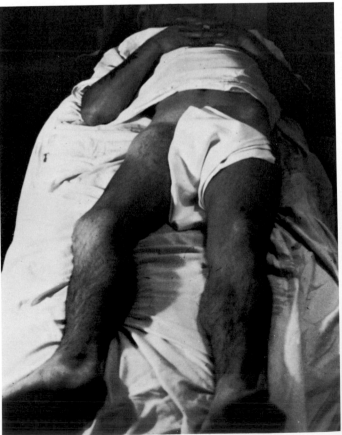

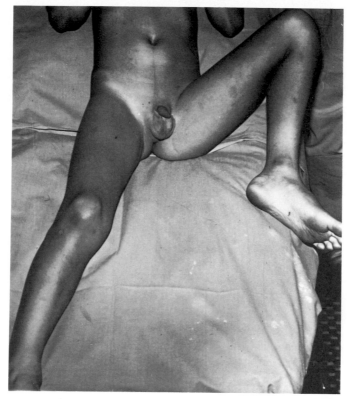

Fig. 1.30 An anterior obturator dislocation, left hip, in a child. Note marked abduction, flexion, and external rotation of the hip.

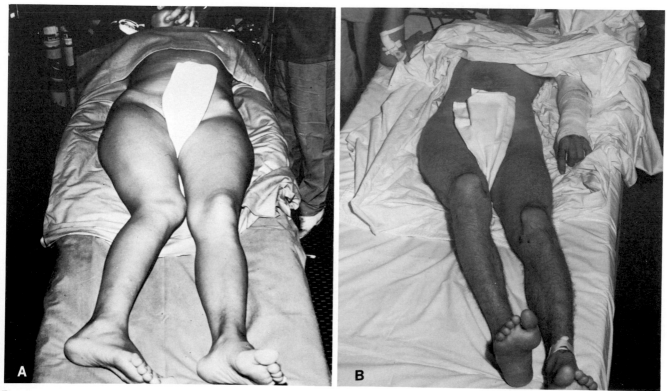

Fig. 1.31 *A* and *B,* posterior dislocation, right hip. Note adduction, internal rotation and shortening.

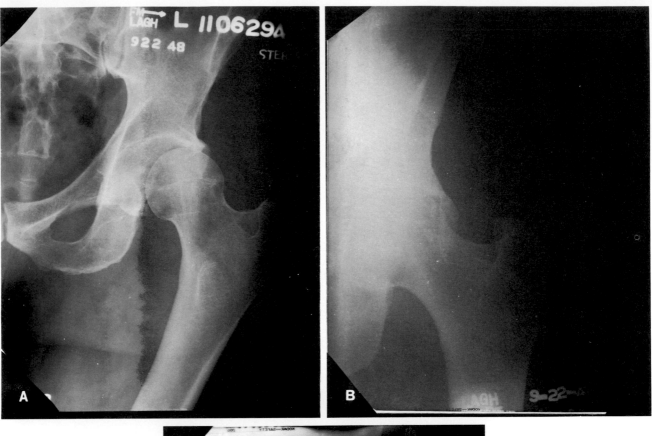

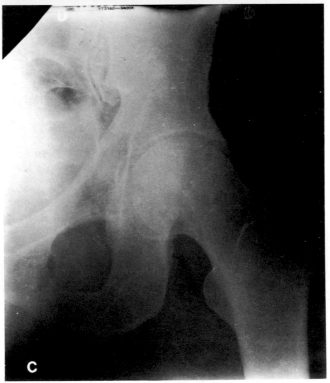

Fig. 1.32 This 53-year-old man was involved in an auto vs. auto accident on September 22, 1948, sustaining a type II posterior dislocation of his left hip. There was also a fracture of the ipsilateral patella but the skin was too contused for immediate open reduction. The result at 12 months was fair with traumatic arthritis. *A,* roentgenogram on day of injury. Note marked adduction of hip and avulsion of posterior superior acetabular rim. *B,* roentgenogram on day of injury after what was thought to be closed reduction under Pentothal and curare anesthesia. The lesser trochanter is still not visible. *C,* two days later the hip was again reduced under a general anesthetic. The lesser trochanter is, now, visualized and the hip is reduced.

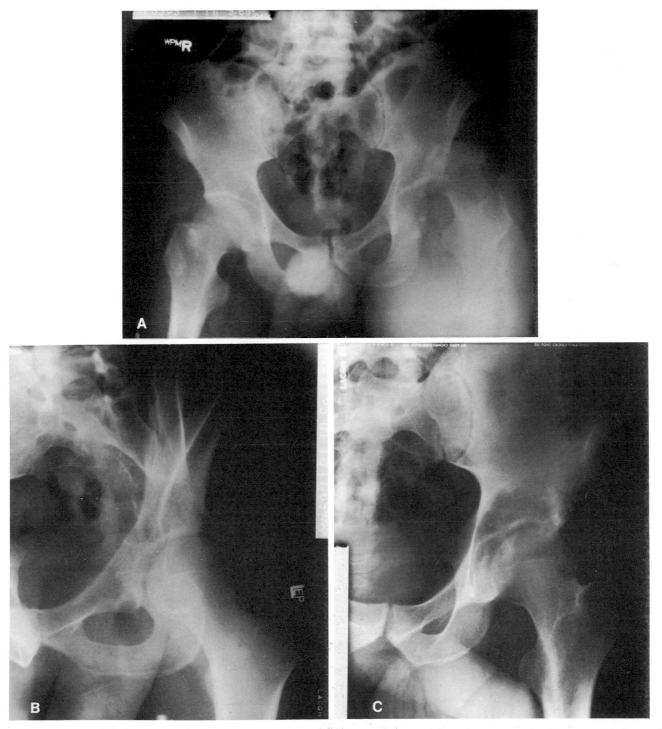

Fig. 1.33 *A,* type III dislocation. AP view reveals posterior dislocation with comminuted posterior rim fragments. *B,* internal oblique view shows posterior acetabular rim fragment and anterior column. *C,* external oblique view shows posterior spine of ilium with apparent reduction of posterior superior acetabular rim.

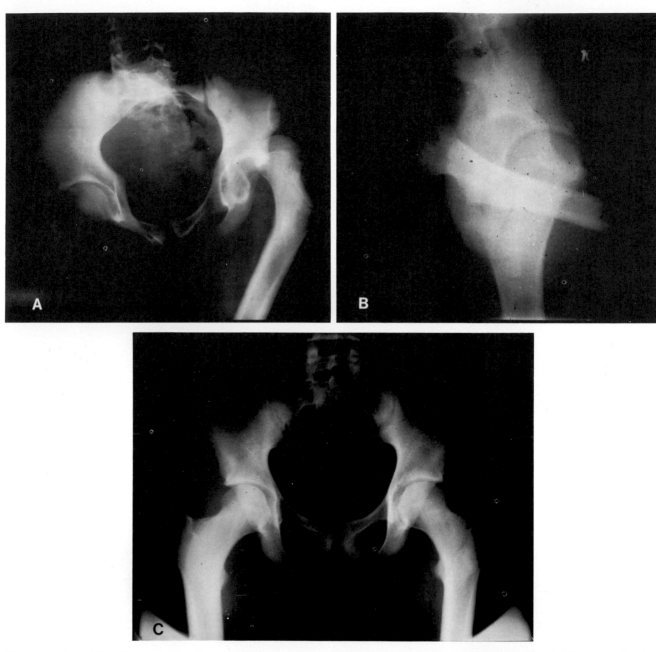

Fig. 1.34 *A* and *B*, a 13-year-old male was struck by a car, sustaining a posterior type I dislocation of the left hip and a fracture of the right greater trochanter. Posterior type I AP, lateral of the left hip. Hip was reduced on the day of injury under a general anesthesia and patient was placed in Russell's traction for 3 weeks. Weight-bearing was started at 4 weeks. *C*, at follow-up 13 years later, there was normal range of hip motion, without complaints, and the roentgenogram was normal.

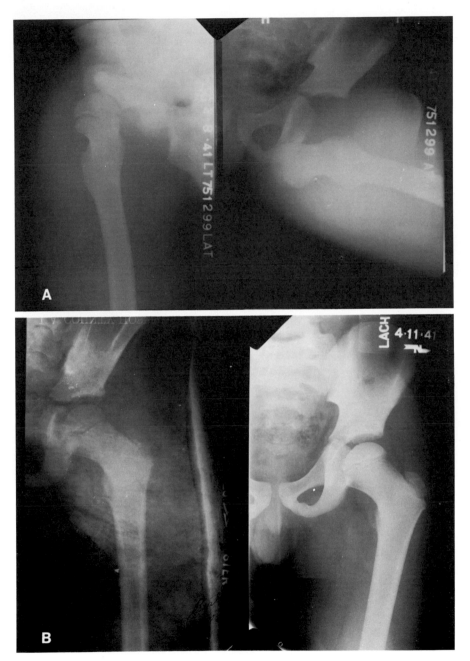

Fig. 1.35 *A,* a 6-year-old boy sustained an anterior dislocation, without fracture, with an excellent result. The patient slipped and fell. The dislocation was reduced on the same day and a spica cast was applied. The patient walked in 3 weeks. *B,* roentgenogram made 2 months later.

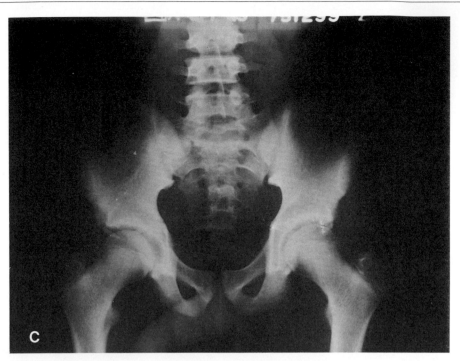

Fig. 1.35   C, follow-up roentgenogram made 8½ years later. There was a normal range of hip motion and the patient had no complaints.

CRITERIA FOR EVALUATING RESULTS

The results were judged independently by roentgenographic and clinical methods. If the two methods disagreed as to result, the case was assigned to the lower of the two grades (Table 1.8).

The roentgenographic rating was based on the following observations:
1. Position: Reduced, not reduced.
2. Cartilaginous joint space: Normal, diminished (mild, moderate, severe).
3. Variations in bone density of head: Mottling, cystic formation, or sequestra.
4. Subchondral irregularities of head.
5. Acetabular sclerosis.
6. Capsular calcification: Mild, moderate, severe.
7. Spur formation: Mild, moderate, severe.

Results were considered to be excellent when there was no change due to trauma (Figs. 1.36 and 1.37), good when there were minimal changes (Figs. 1.38 and 1.39), fair when changes were moderate (Figs. 1.40 and 1.41), and poor when changes were severe (Figs. 1.42 and 1.43).

The clinical criteria for the evaluation of results are summarized in Table 1.9.

With respect to subjective findings, patients who had *no pain* were considered to have excellent or good results. A patient with a good result, however, might have a sense of stiffness after long sitting. Patients were considered to have a fair result if they had some pain but not to an incapacitating degree, even if they had to change to a less arduous occupation than before. In those patients with poor results the pain was considered disabling even if the patient was only partially incapacitated. Thus, a housewife able to do her cleaning and cooking adequately, but requiring frequent rest or a crutch, was considered to have a poor result.

Table 1.8
Roentgenographic Criteria for Evaluating Results

Excellent (normal)
  All of the following:
  1. Normal relationship between head and acetabulum
  2. Normal articular cartilaginous space
  3. Normal density head of femur
  4. No spur formation
  5. No calcification in capsule
Good (minimal changes)
  1. Normal relationship between head and acetabulum
  2. Minimal narrowing of cartilaginous space
  3. Minimal deossification
  4. Minimal spur formation
  5. Minimal capsular calcification
Fair (moderate changes)
  1. Normal relationship between head and acetabulum
  Any one or more of the following:
  2. Moderate narrowing of cartilaginous space
  3. Mottling of head, areas of sclerosis and decreased density
  4. Moderate spur formation
  5. Moderate to severe capsular calcification
  6. Depression of subchondral cortex of the femoral head
Poor (severe changes)
  1. Almost complete obliteration of cartilaginous space
  2. Relative increase in density of femoral head
  3. Subchondral cyst formation
  4. Formation of sequestra
  5. Gross deformity of femoral head
  6. Severe spur formation
  7. Acetabular sclerosis

Table 1.9
Clinical Criteria for Evaluating Results

Excellent (all of the following)
  1. No pain
  2. Full range of hip motion
  3. No limp
  4. No roentgenographic evidence of progressive changes
Good
  1. No pain
  2. Free motion (75% of normal hip)
  3. No more than a slight limp
  4. Minimal roentgenographic changes
Fair (any one or more of the following)
1. Pain, but not disabling
2. Limited motion of hip; no adduction deformity
3. Moderate limp
4. Moderately severe roentgenographic changes
Poor (any one or more of the following)
  1. Disabling pain
  2. Marked limitation of motion or adduction deformity
  3. Redislocation
  4. Progressive roentgenographic changes

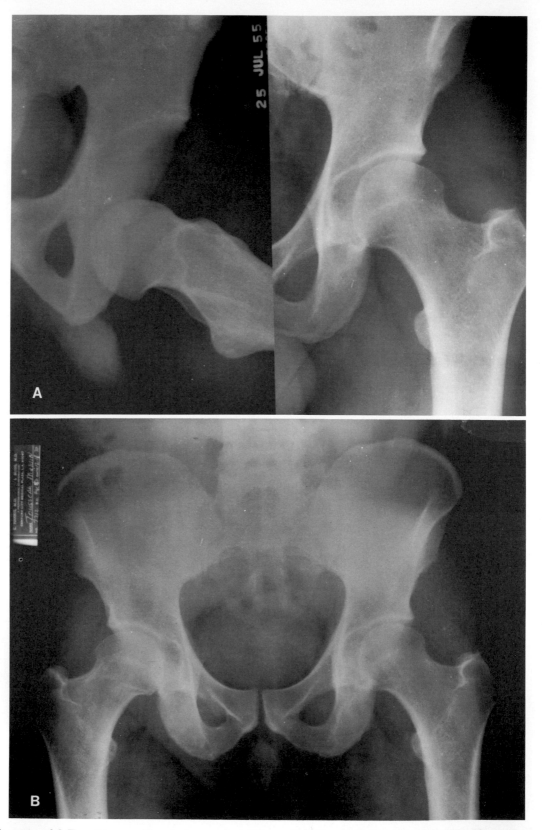

Fig. 1.36 *A,* patient M. T., a 30-year-old male in an automobile accident in which the car turned over. The patient sustained an anterior dislocation of the left hip. The result 19 years later was rated excellent. Roentgenograms taken before and after reduction. The dislocation was reduced closed, under general anesthesia, within a few hours of injury in a small mountain town in Montana. He started weight bearing the same day. *B,* roentgenogram made at follow-up. The joint space is normal. The patient had normal range of hip motion without any complaints. (From Epstein, H. C.: Traumatic anterior and simple posterior dislocations of the hip in adults and chidren. In *The American Academy of Orthopaedic Surgeons: Instructional Course Lectures,* vol. 22. The C. V. Mosby Co., St. Louis, 1973. Reproduced with permission.)

36

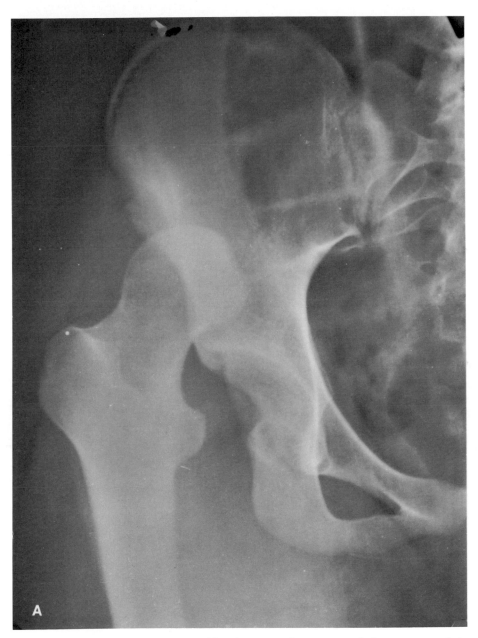

Fig. 1.37 *A,* Patient R. M., a 16-year-old girl, sustained a posterior dislocation, type I, in a collision between an automobile and a freight train. The result was excellent. *A,* roentgenogram made on the day of injury.

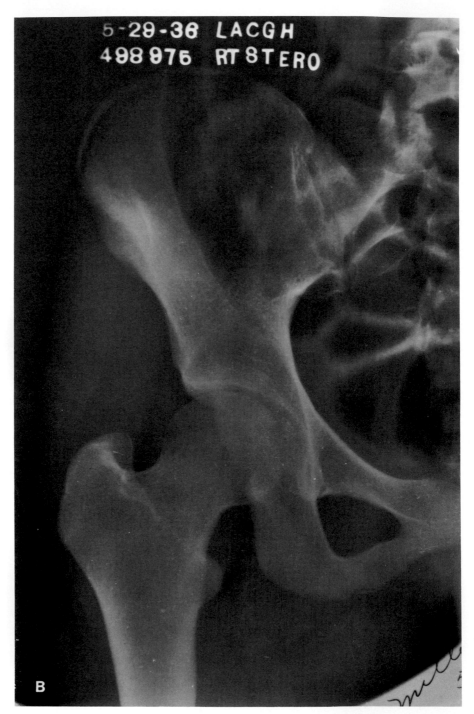

Fig. 1.37 *B,* roentgenogram made on the same day of injury after reduction. The period of bed rest was 3 weeks and the patient walked after 7 weeks.

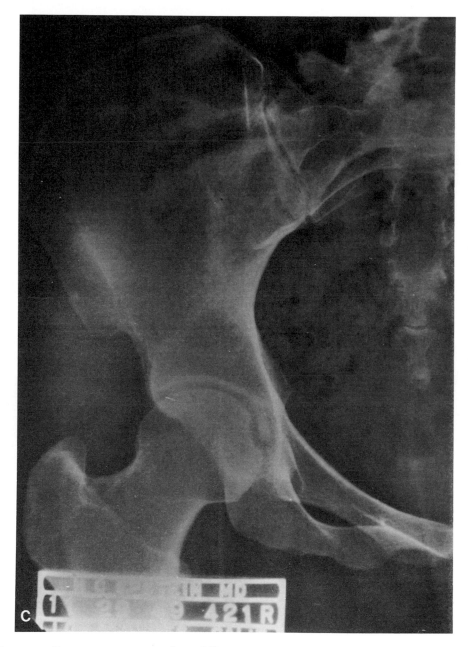

Fig. 1.37 C, roentgenogram made at follow-up examination, 13 years and 1 month later. There is an ununited fragment at the site of the attachment of the ligamentum teres. The range of hip motion was normal and the patient had no complaints.

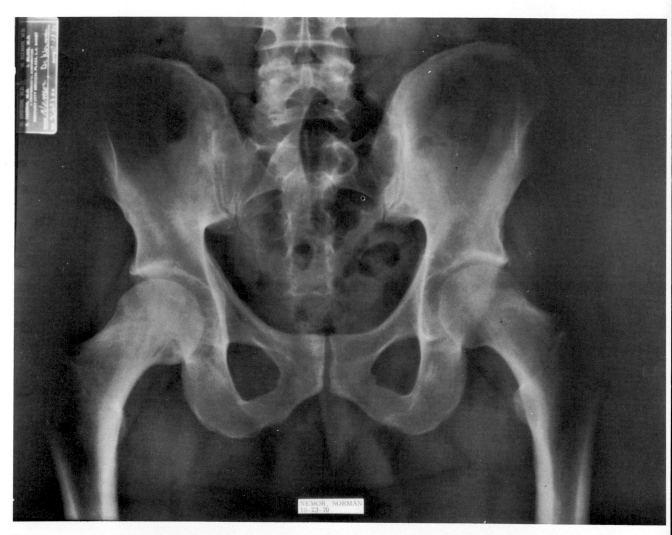

Fig. 1.38　A 23-year-old male dislocated his left hip in a sledding accident. The result, 27 years later, is good. Roentgenogram made at follow-up of a simple type I dislocation. The hip was reduced the day of injury with the patient at bed rest for 1 week only. He started to walk by the 3rd week. The roentgenogram is normal but there is minimal restriction of motion of the left hip. He had no complaints of pain or discomfort.

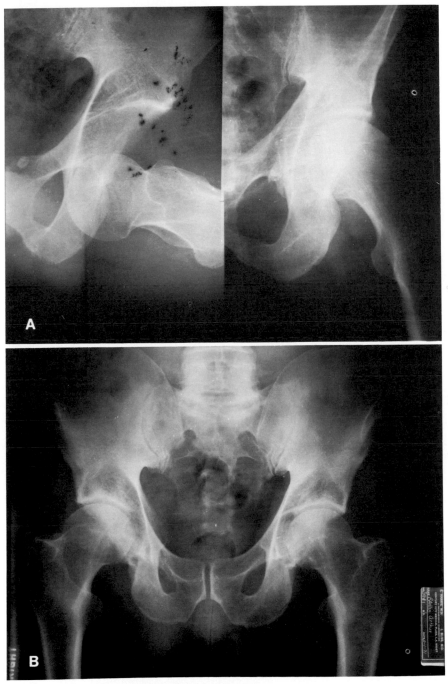

Fig. 1.39 A 42-year-old man in an auto accident sustained this anterior dislocation of his left hip. There was also a cerebral concussion. The result 9 nine years later was good. *A,* the obturator dislocation was reduced closed on the day of injury under general anesthesia. Traction was maintained for 2 weeks, then no weight-bearing with crutches and weight-bearing started by 5th week. *B,* nine years after injury there is a minimal restriction of internal and external rotation of the left hip. The patient has no pain and plays golf, carrying his own golf bag. The roentgenogram appears normal.

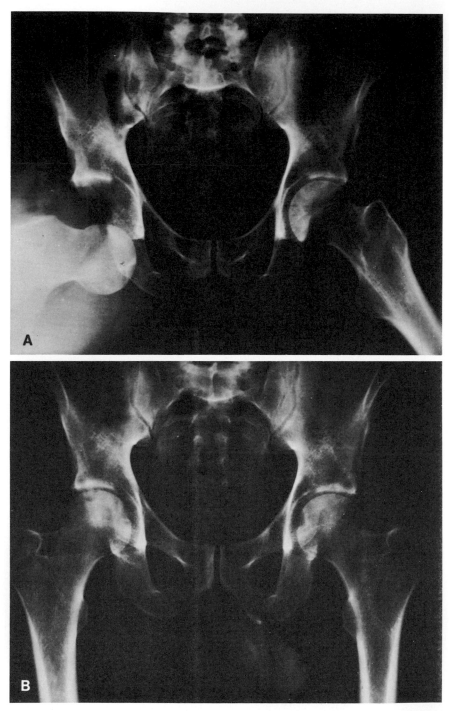

Fig. 1.40 *A,* a 32-year-old man a (passenger) was thrown out of a small car in an auto accident, sustaining this obturator dislocation. *B,* reduction was performed the day of injury. Note the defect in the femoral head.

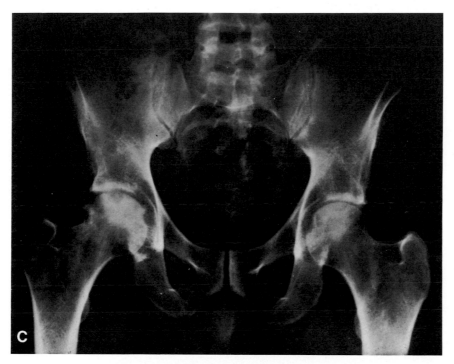

Fig. 1.40 C, at 2½ years after injury, anteroposterior roentgenograms reveal traumatic arthritis, although it looks like avascular necrosis. There are areas of increased and decreased densities in the femoral head with narrowing of the joint space and spur formation of the neck, superiorly and inferiorly. Patient had 1½ inches of atrophy of the right thigh, moderate limitation of hip motion, and intermittent episodes of hip pain. Result is rated fair.

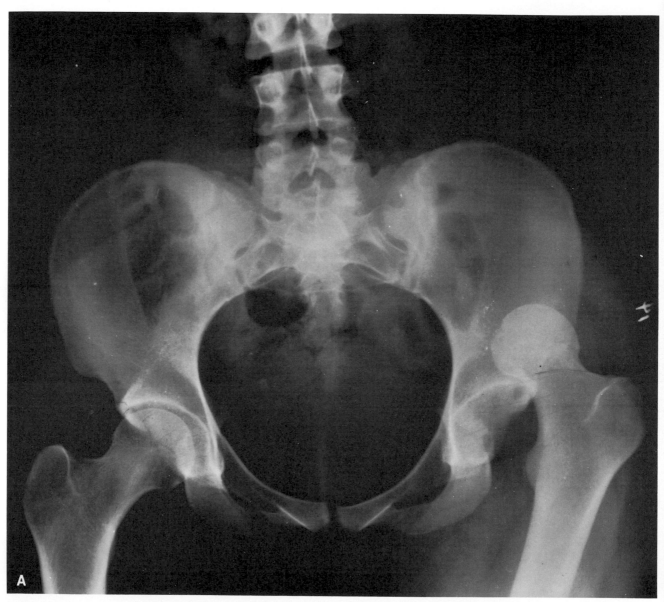

Fig. 1.41   *A,* a 19-year-old female dislocated her left hip in an automobile accident; the left knee striking the dashboard. The result 14 years later is fair.

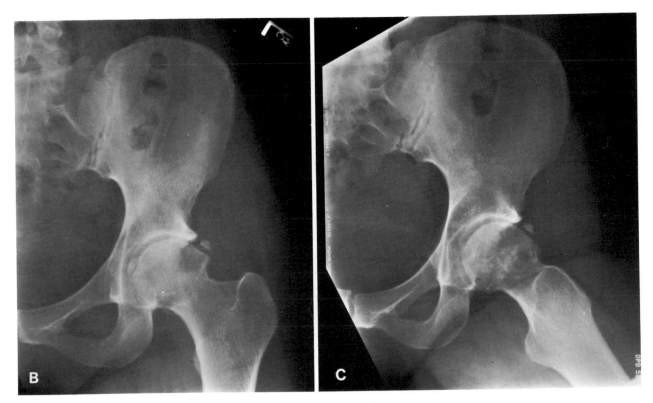

Fig. 1.41 *B,* roentgenogram of a simple dislocation with a chip fracture. Reduction was accomplished the day of injury under general anesthesia. The patient was placed in Russell traction for 3 weeks and then started weight-bearing. *C,* follow-up roentgenogram shows a small spur lying over the superior portion of the head of the femur. At times the patient has a sensation of a "catch" in the hip joint. The spur may be acting as a loose body on certain motions of the hip. The range of hip motion is normal. Surgery has been advised for removal of the loose body if there are symptoms of discomfort and pain.

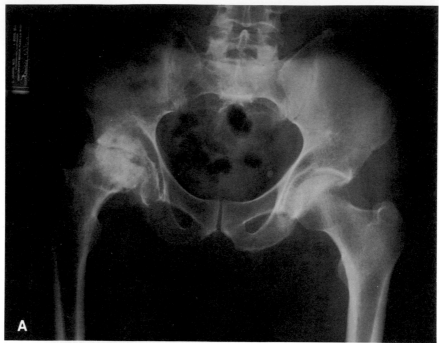

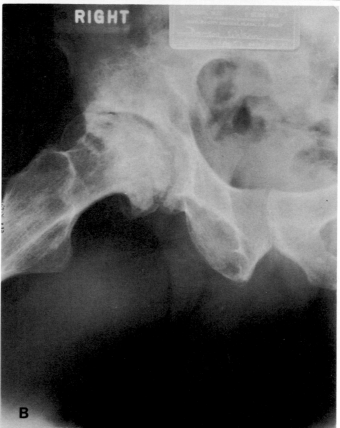

Fig. 1.42 R. W., a 47-year-old male, slipped and fell downstairs, dislocating the right hip. The result, 10 years later, was poor with avascular necrosis (type I). *A,* roentgenogram made at follow-up reveals advanced changes of avascular necrosis with irregularity, widening of the femoral head, and sclerotic changes in both the femoral and acetabular portions of the hip joint. *B,* there are large osteophytes and cystic changes. The hip was easily reduced on the day of injury under general anesthesia. He was kept in traction for 5 weeks and then gradually started to bear weight. The patient stated he has had pain in the hip since he started to walk. On examination there is considerable pain and marked limitation of motion and the patient wants some procedure performed for relief.

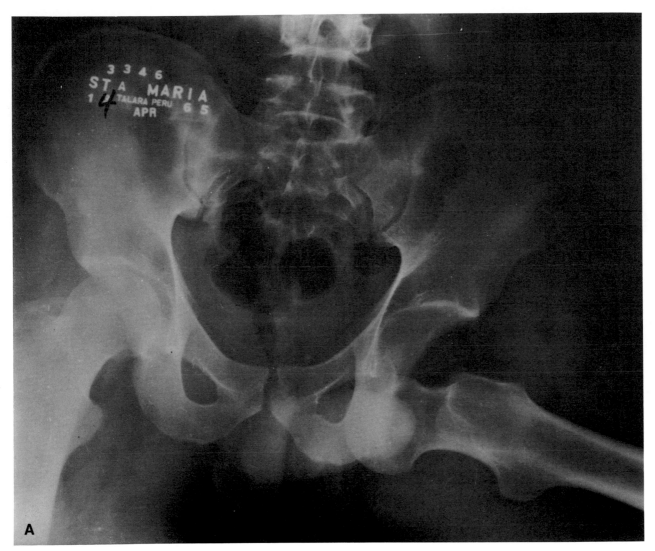

Fig. 1.43 *A*, patient E. K., a 25-year-old male, sustained an anterior dislocation of the left hip. He developed avascular necrosis and the result was rated poor. The dislocation occurred on board a fishing boat when a hopper, weighing one-half ton, fell on the patient pinning him to the floor. The hip was in extreme abduction and a mattress was placed under the hip for support.

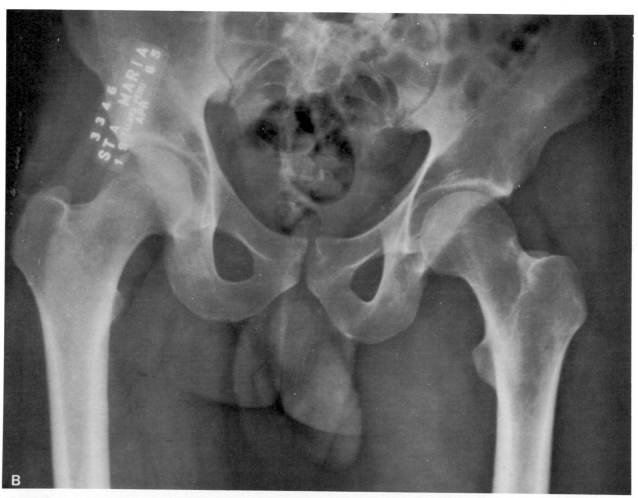

Fig. 1.43 *B*, roentgenogram shows reduction of the hip performed 18 hours after injury when the ship landed in Lima, Peru. The patient was hospitalized and traction was applied for 30 days; then he started weight-bearing.

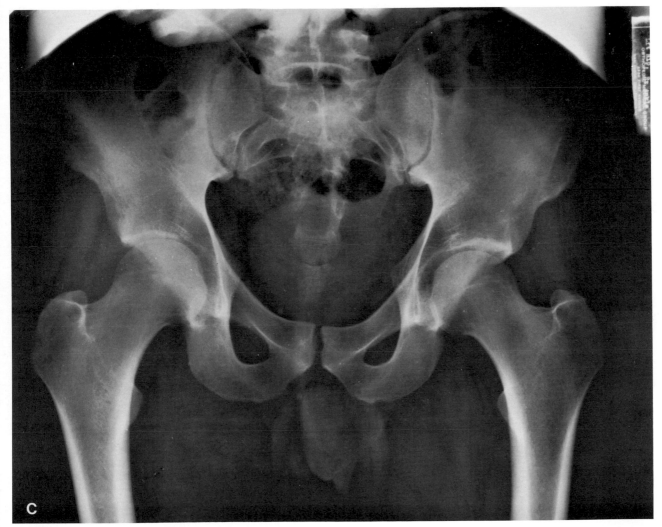

Fig. 1.43 C, roentgenogram made 2 months after injury. There is no definite evidence of avascular necrosis although the patient complained of pain on any motion of the hip.

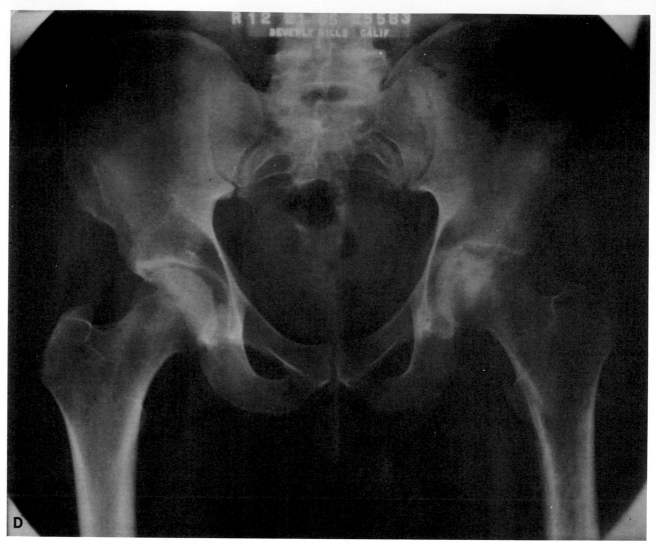

Fig. 1.43   *D,* roentgenogram made 8 months after injury. There is definite evidence of avascular necrosis with irregularity of the weight-bearing portion of the femoral head with collapse. The patient subsequently had a fusion of the hip.

Objectively, those hips with normal physical findings were classified as excellent, whereas those with some restriction of motion, but without muscle spasm or deformity, were classified as good. Some patients with a good result had a slight limp after fast walking or gave a history of limp upon fatigue. Patients with significant limitation of motion but no adduction deformity were considered to have a fair result; in these patients muscle spasm usually could be elicited by forcing motions at their extremes; a limp was usually present. The findings in the poor results were muscle spasm with severe restriction of motion, adduction deformity, and limp.

CHAPTER
2

POSTERIOR TYPE I DISLOCATIONS

There were 17 excellent (Figs. 2.1 A–C; 2.2A–C) and 70 good results (Figs. 2.3; 2.4 A, B) in the 134 dislocated hips, a 65% incidence of excellent-good; the unsatisfactory results were 20, fair (Figs. 2.5A, 2.8A–C) and 27 with poor results (Figs. 2.7A–D; 2.8A–C), a 35 % incidence (Table 2.1).

The results of the long-term follow-up obtained in this adult series of 134 indicates that "simple" type I dislocations are not so simple and in the prognoses one would have to consider that approximately one-third of these patients will have some future disability. In the 1950 series,[100] out of a total of 30 cases with posterior type I dislocations, two-thirds had excellent or good results and one-third had fair or poor results.

There were 12 type I dislocations in patients 16 years of age who were followed for 2 to 13 years (Fig. 1.37A–C), with excellent or good results in 11 and a fair result in one. These have been included in the adult series.

In six cases of posterior type I dislocations there was an insignificant chip fracture about the acetabululm. Results were good in three cases, fair in two, and poor in one. This small series indicates that fragments not visible by roentgenogram may be dislodged from the acetabulum or the femoral head and left in the hip joint, resulting in a guarded prognosis for this type of injury (Fig. 2.9A, B).

In those cases with dislocations and fractures of the pelvis the prognosis should also remain guarded. Of eight such injuries the results were good in three cases, fair in two, and poor in two (Figs. 2.10A–C; 2.11A, B). Follow-up was insufficient in one case.

There were no excellent results but three good results (Fig. 2.12A–C)in cases in which more than one reduction was done (Table 2.2). One irreducible hip had an open reduction the day of injury with a good result (Fig. 2.13A–C). One irreducible hip was scheduled for an open reduction but the patient signed out against consent. Two months later, at another hospital, the patient died during an attempt at open reduction. One other case in which the hip was never reduced had a poor result and in one other case the hip was irreducible by closed method, followed 2½ months later by an open reduction with a poor result.

In a previous report, Thompson and Epstein,[100] stated there were no excellent or good results in those dislocations requiring two or more reductions or in those not reduced. It is obvious that one reduction is better for the patient than adding trauma on trauma. The lack of success in an early attempt at closed reduction suggests that open reduction may be necessary in such cases.

Table 2.1
Results—Posterior Type I Dislocations[a]

Excellent	Good	Fair	Poor	Total	Percentage of excellent-good results
17	70[b]	20	27	134	65

[a] Average follow-up, 77.8 months.
[b] One hip irreducible closed; opened day of injury. Good, 23 years.

Table 2.2
Number of Closed Reductions Compared with Outcome for 134 Type Dislocations

One reduction				Two or more reductions				Not reduced			
Excellent	Good	Fair	Poor	Excellent	Good	Fair	Poor	Excellent	Good	Fair	Poor
17	66	18	21	0	3	2	4[a]	0	1[b]	0	2[c]

[a] One reduced 2 weeks after injury and one irreducible with open surgery 2½ months later.
[b] Irreducible closed; then opened day of injury with good results.
[c] One irreducible and one was never reduced.

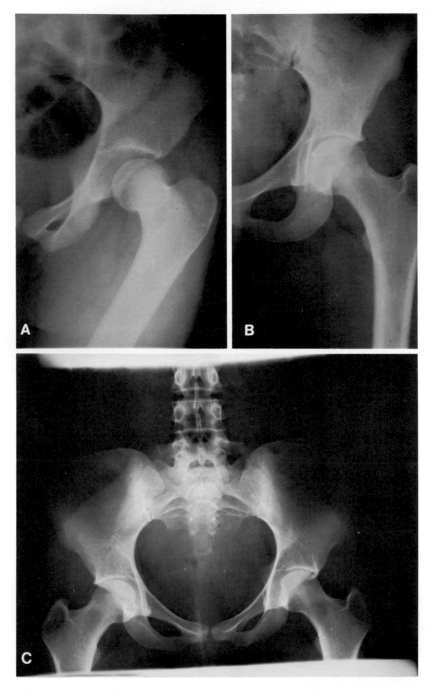

Fig. 2.1 T. F., a 17-year-old girl, a passenger in an automobile collision, was thrown from the back seat and sustained a simple posterior dislocation of the left hip. The result, 62 months later, was excellent. *A,* roentgenogram reveals a posterior dislocation without fracture. *B,* reduction was accomplished the day of injury under morphine sulfate by the Allis method. Russell traction followed for 3 weeks and weight-bearing started at 4 weeks. *C,* at follow-up, 62 months later, there were no complaints and the roentgenogram was normal.

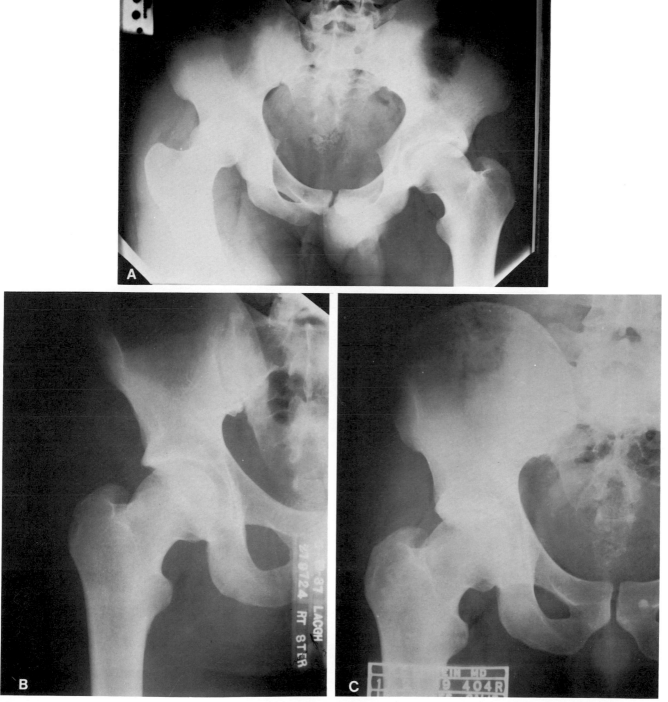

Fig. 2.2 J. C., a 22-year-old male, sustained a posterior type I dislocation of the right hip when his automobile overturned. A peroneal palsy returned to normal in 6 months. The result, $12\frac{1}{2}$ years later, was excellent. *A*, roentgenogram shows a simple posterior dislocation of the right hip, *B*, roentgenogram made after reduction. The hip was reduced by the Stimson method on the day of injury. Buck's traction was maintained for 3 weeks and then weight-bearing was started. *C*, roentgenogram made at follow-up was normal. The patient had normal range of hip motions, without complaints.

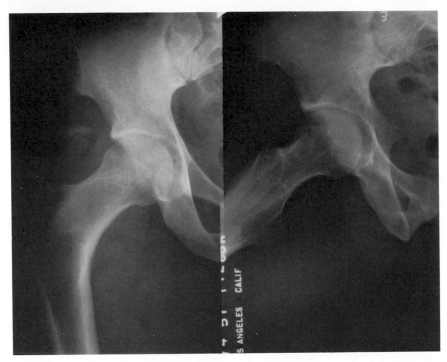

Fig. 2.3   H. R., a 39-year-old male with a posterior type I dislocation of the right hip sustained in an automobile vs. automobile accident. The result, 19 years later, is good. Anteroposterior and lateral rotengenograms of the right hip made at the last follow-up. Reduction was performed at another hospital on the day of injury. The method of reduction was not specified. Traction was maintained for 3 weeks and weight-bearing started at 4 months. The roentgenograms appear to be normal. The patient was given a rating of good rather than excellent, because there was 10° limitation of internal and external rotation of the hip. (From Epstein, H. C.: Traumatic anterior and simple posterior dislocations of the hip in adults and children. In *The American Academy of Orthopaedic Surgeons: Instructional Course Lectures,* vol. 22. The C. V. Mosby Co., St. Louis, 1973. Reproduced with permission.)

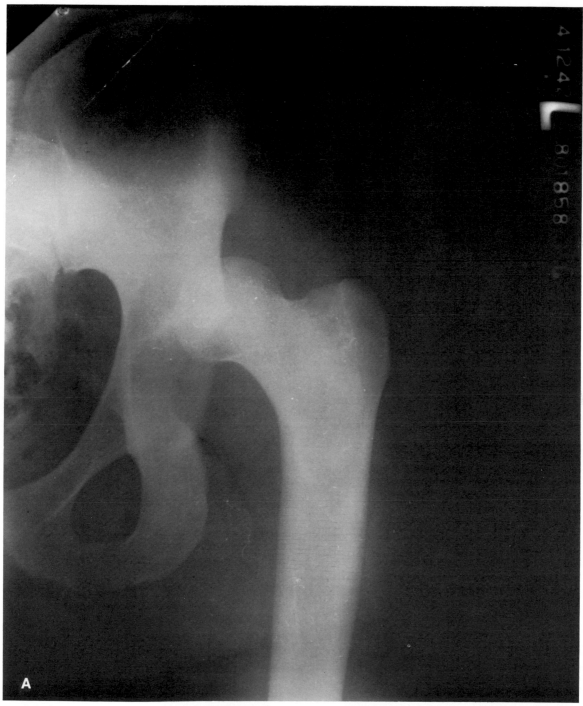

Fig. 2.4 *A*, patient G. J., a 20-year-old male, sustained a left posterior dislocation, type I. The result was good. Roentgenogram made on the day of injury. The patient was in an automobile which crashed into a train. The dislocation was reduced on the same day. Traction was applied for 10 days and the patient walked after 6 weeks.

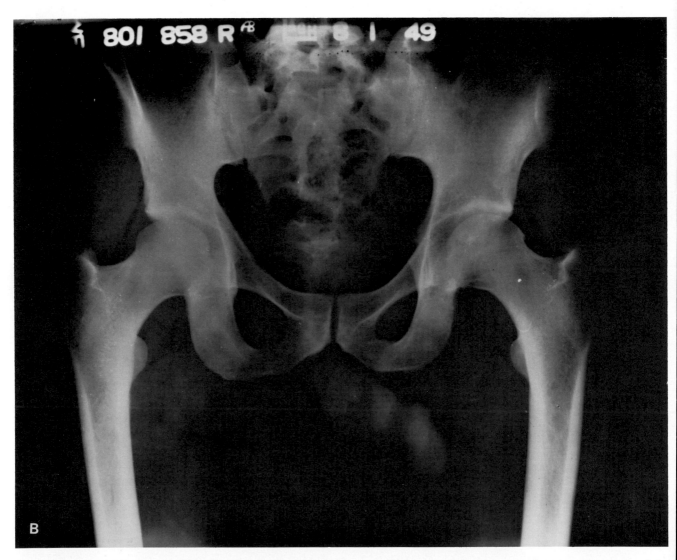

Fig. 2.4 *B*, roentgenogram made 7 years and 4 months later. There is minimal spur formation at the superior margin of the head and neck. The patient had no pain but felt discomfort after sitting and there was slight limitation of hip motion. (*A* and *B*, from Epstein, H. C.: Traumatic anterior and simple posterior dislocations of the hip in adults and children. In *The American Academy of Orthopaedic Surgeons: Instructional Course Lectures,* vol. 22. The C. V. Mosby Co., St. Louis, 1973. Reproduced with permission.)

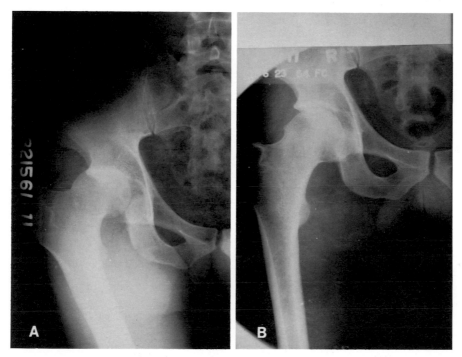

Fig. 2.5   H. B., 25-year-old motorcyclist, dislocated his right hip when he struck a parked car. Twenty months later the result was rated good with minimal traumatic arthritis. At 10 years, the result was rated fair. *A,* roentgenogram of a posterior type I dislocation. The hip was reduced under general anesthesia the day of injury and a spica cast was applied for 3 weeks. Weight-bearing started at 4 weeks. *B,* there is minimal spur formation at the superior border of the junction of the head and neck with minimal narrowing of the joint space. The range of motion is normal and the patient had no complaints.

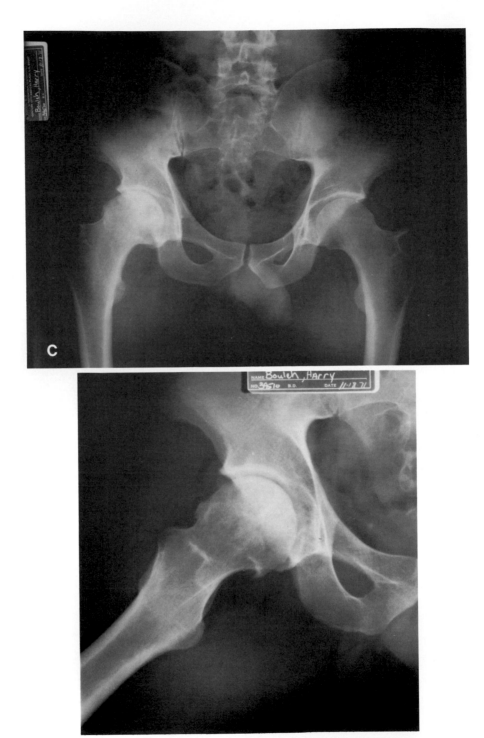

Fig. 2.5   C, anterior-posterior and lateral roentgenograms taken 10 years after injury. There is more narrowing of the hip joint with more prominent osteophytes at the superior and inferior borders of the head and neck. The patient has moderate pain but continues to work.

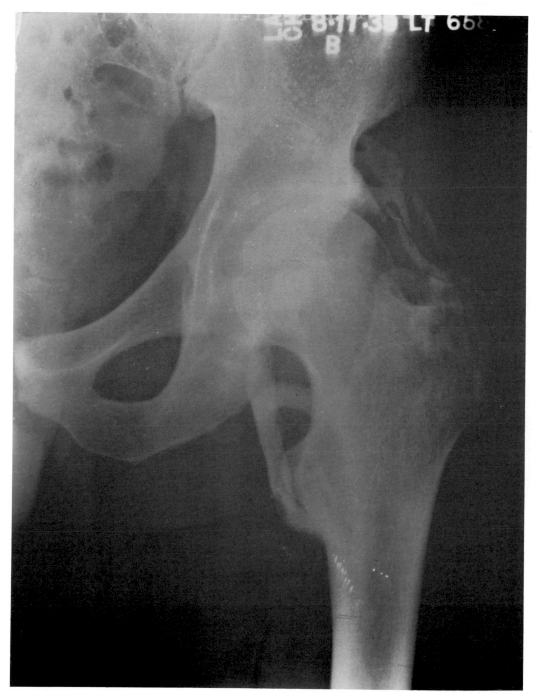

Fig. 2.6 H. C., 21 years old, was injured in an automobile accident and entered the hospital 12 days postinjury. The roentgenogram shows a reduced posterior type I dislocation which later had a fair result. Three attempts at reduction were made within 3 days. The period of follow-up was 5 months. There was extensive myositis ossificans. (From Epstein, H. C.: Traumatic anterior and simple posterior dislocations of the hip in adults and children. In *The American Academy of Orthopaedic Surgeons: Instructional Course Lectures,* vol. 22. The C. V. Mosby Co., St. Louis, 1973. Reproduced with permission.)

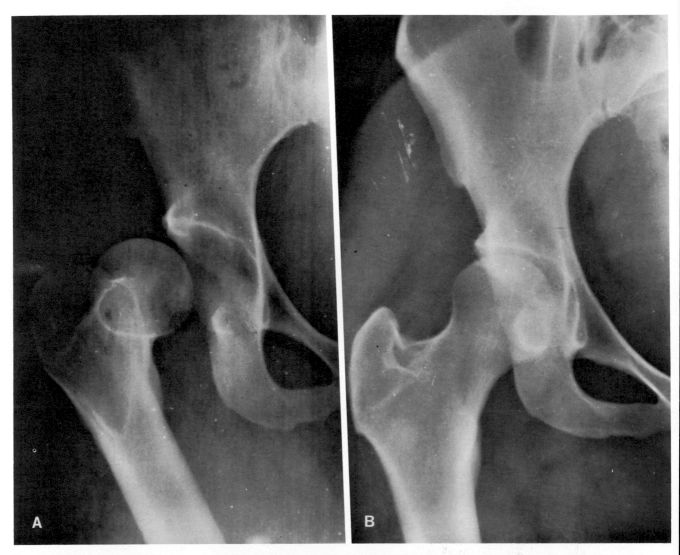

Fig. 2.7   V. T., a 22-year-old woman, sustained a simple dislocation of the right hip. The result, 58 months later, was rated poor with avascular necrosis. *A,* roentgenogram made the day of injury by injury before reduction. *B,* the hip was reduced closed the day of injury by the Allis method under iv Demerol. The patient was kept in Russell traction for 3 months and then started weight-bearing. The patient also had a fracture of the second and third lumbar vertebrae and a fracture of the right lateral malleolus. She developed mumps while in the hospital.

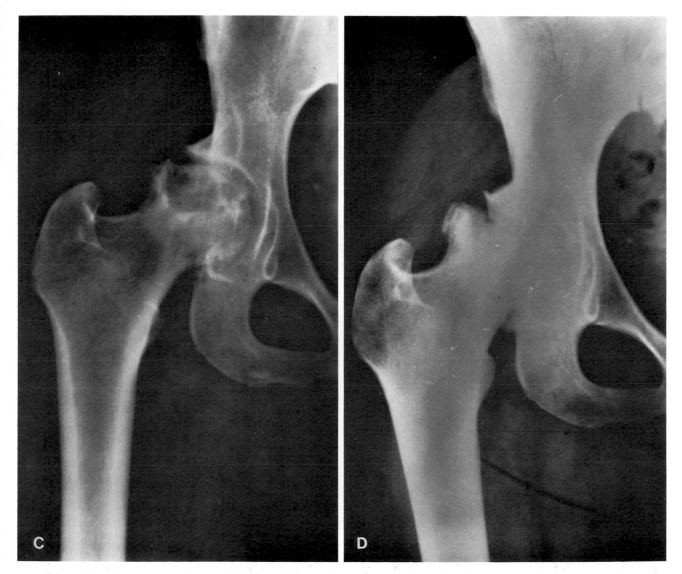

Fig. 2.7 *C,* three years later there is early collapse of the head of the femur with avascular necrosis. *D,* roentgenogram shows further collapse of the femoral head with disintegration of the hip joint. Although the patient has pain and limitation of motion she does not want any other procedures performed at the present time. (*A–C* from Epstein, H. C.: Traumatic anterior and simple posterior dislocations of the hip in adults and children. In *The American Academy of Orthopaedic Surgeons: Instructional Course Lectures,* vol. 22. The C. V. Mosby Co., St. Louis, 1973. Reproduced with permission.)

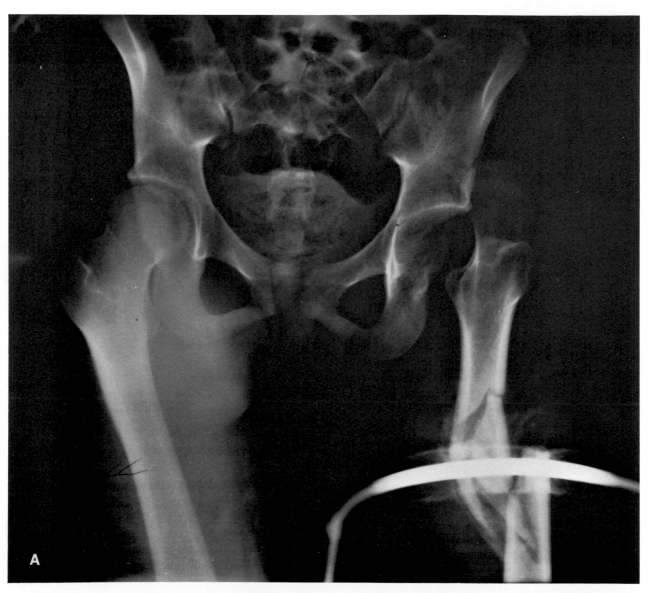

Fig. 2.8 C. D., an 18-year-old female, in an automobile accident, sustained a posterior dislocation of the left hip with a fracture of the ipsilateral femur and a severe laceration of her liver (type I). *A*, there was an unsuccessful attempt at closed reduction at the time the patient had a repair for the laceration of the liver. She was then treated in traction.

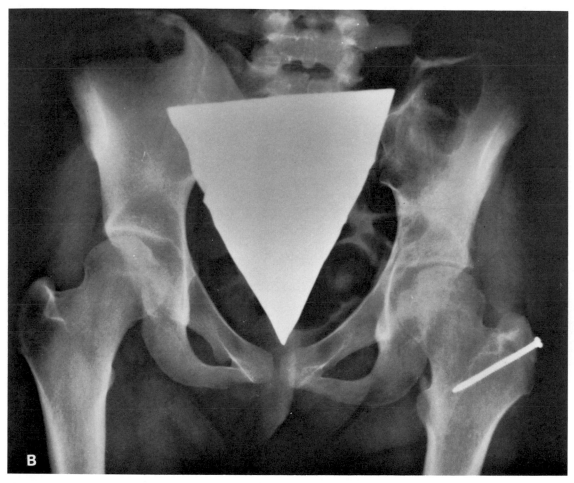

Fig. 2.8 *B*, open reduction was performed 2½ months after injury and later a derotational osteotomy was performed to correct the femoral fracture. Note the areas of increased and decreased densities throughout the femoral head, with a normal cartilaginous joint space.

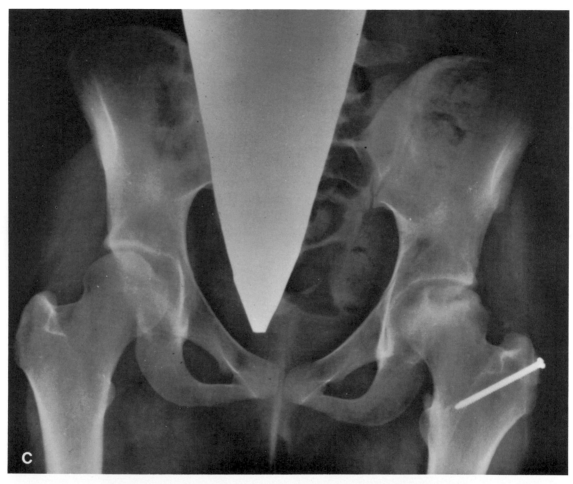

Fig. 2.8 *C,* six months following open reduction there is definite avascular necrosis with collapse of the femoral head. The patient has moderate restriction of hip motion and pain, with a poor result. (*A–C* from Epstein, H. C.: Traumatic anterior and simple posterior dislocations of the hip in adults and children. In *The American Academy of Orthopaedic Surgeons: Instructional Course Lectures,* vol. 22. The C. V. Mosby Co., St. Louis, 1973. Reproduced with permission.)

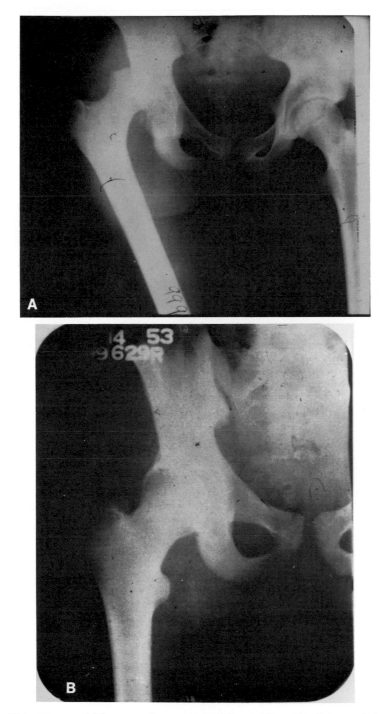

Fig. 2.9 This 14-year-old boy was in an automobile accident. He dislocated the right hip with a chip fracture of the posterior rim of the acetabulum. The result was rated good, 5 years later. *A*, the hip was reduced by closed manipulation (Allis method) under general anesthesia on the day of injury. Russell traction was maintained for 4 weeks and then patient started to bear weight. *B*, there is minimal restriction of range of motion. He has no complaints of pain.

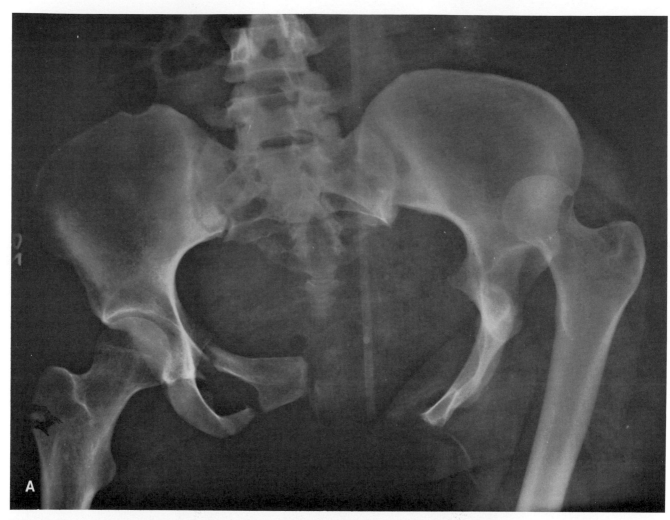

Fig. 2.10   F. F., a 28-year-old woman struck by an automobile. She sustained a posterior dislocated hip with a fractured pelvis. The result, 10 months later, is rated as fair. *A,* roentgenogram shows a dislocation of the left hip with a severe fracture of the pelvis.

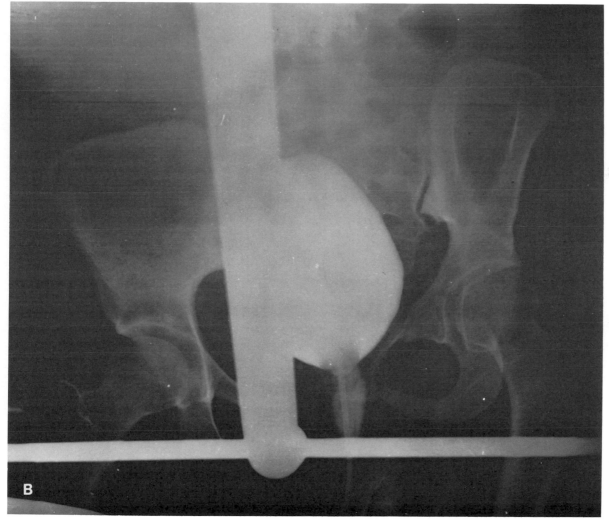

Fig. 2.10 *B,* postreduction was accomplished the same day by 15 minutes of steady pull in line of the deformity under general anesthesia. Traction was maintained for 2½ weeks and weight-bearing was started at 3 months.

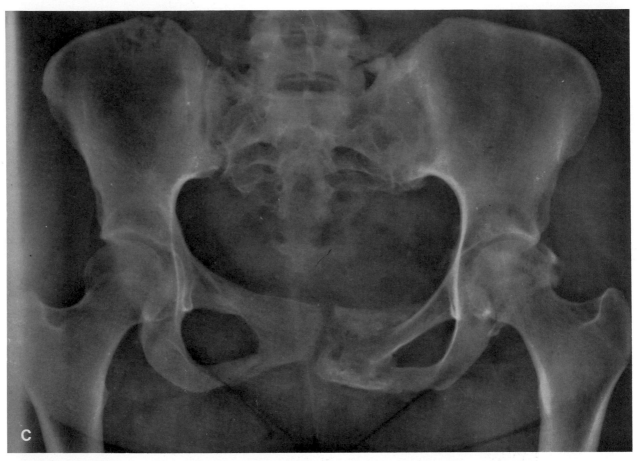

Fig. 2.10 *C*, roentgenogram shows areas of increased and decreased densities throughout the femoral head and moderate narrowing of the hip joint. The separation of the symphysis pubis has been reduced and the pubic fractures are well healed. There is soft tissue calcification. The patient had pain and limitation of motion of the hip.

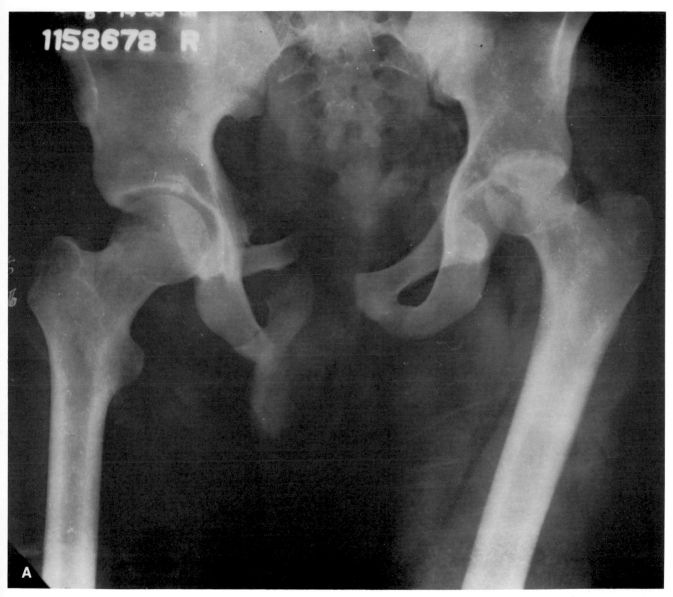

Fig. 2.11 M. F., an 18-year-old male, sustained a posterior dislocation in an automobile accident with fractures of both pubic rami and separation of the symphysis pubis. At follow-up, 40 months later, the result is rated poor (type I). *A*, the hip was easily reduced under general anesthesia at the first attempt. Patient was then transferred to private care.

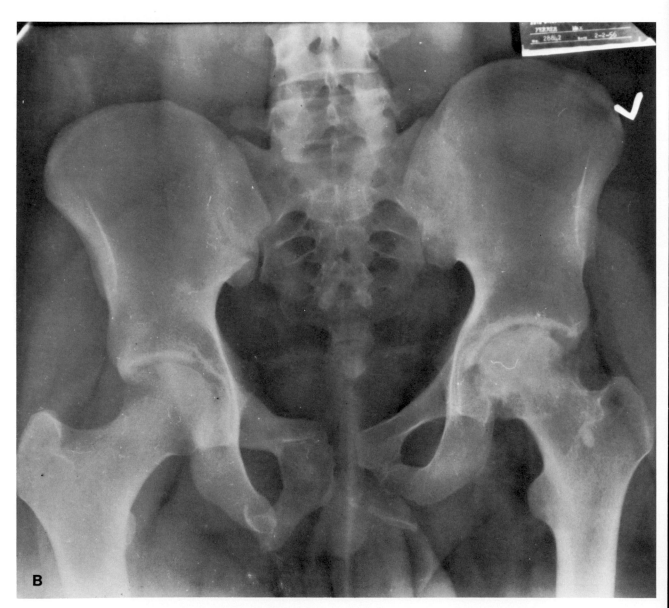

Fig. 2.11   *B,* roentgenogram shows avascular necrosis of the femoral head 40 months after injury.

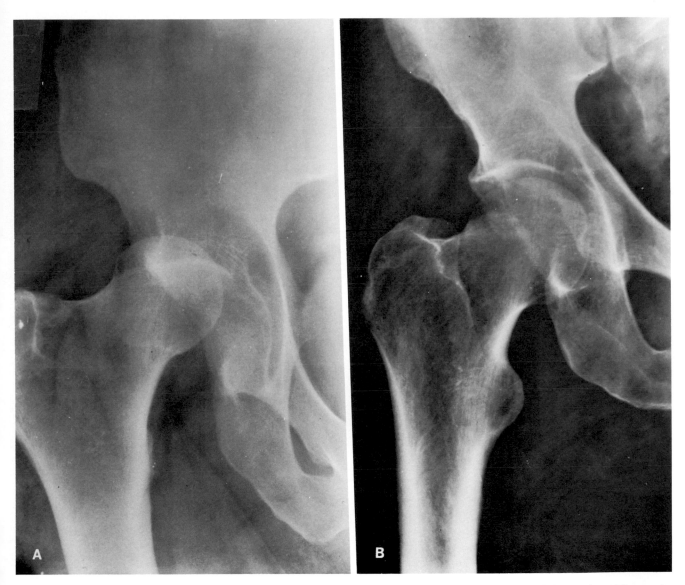

Fig. 2.12 C. P., a blind, 44-year-old male, sustained a type I dislocation of the right hip in an automobile accident. The result was good 5 years later. *A*, roentgenogram shows a type I dislocation. Two attempts at reduction under iv Demerol were unsuccessful. The hip was successfully reduced on the third attempt by the Allis maneuver. *B*, roentgenogram made after reduction. The patient was placed in Russell traction for 1 month and he walked in 2 months.

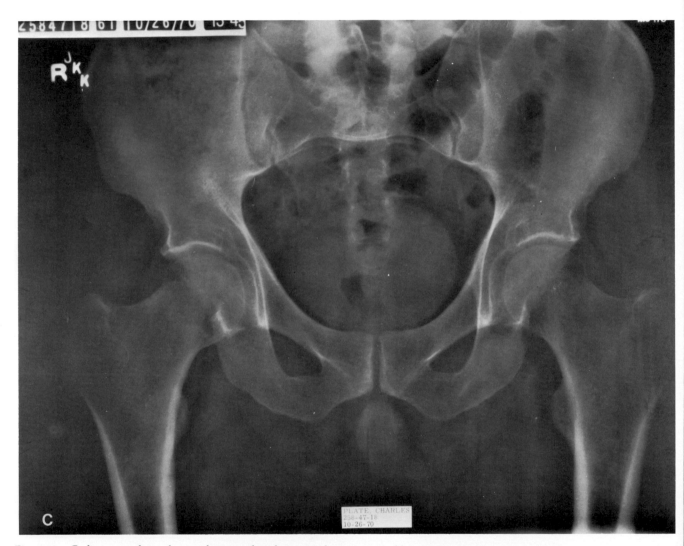

Fig. 2.12 C, five years later the result is good with minimal restriction of hip motions and normal roentgenogram.

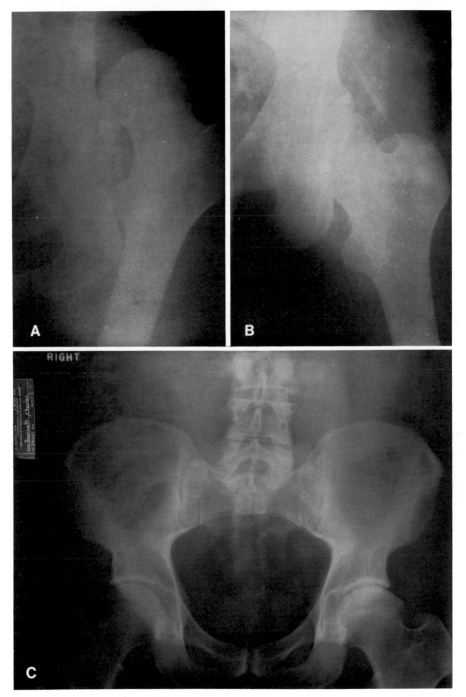

Fig. 2.13 C. B., a 23-year-old male, sustained a simple posterior dislocation of the left hip in September 1950 in a truck vs. cable tower accident. The force of impact drove the truck engine against the patient's left foot, driving it backward. At 21½ years later the result is good. *A,* an attempt at closed reduction under general anesthesia using the Allis maneuver was unsuccessful. *B,* an immediate open reduction using a posterior approach was performed the day of injury. At surgery the entire acetabular labrum was detached and acted as a bowstring across the joint, preventing relocation of the hip. After the entire labrum was removed the hip reduced easily. Weight-bearing was started at 6 weeks after Russell traction. *C,* roentgenogram at follow-up, 21½ years after injury. Patient stated he has never had any pain or discomfort in the left hip. Motion of the hip was normal except for 10° limitation of external and internal rotation. Although the joint space is normal, the left femoral head looks different from that of the right.

METHOD OF REDUCTION

In the majority of cases in this series, the Allis method was used for closed reduction (Fig. 2.14*A–D*). General principles of reduction are traction in the line of deformity, flexion, restoration of alignment, and apposition in the absence of muscle spasm. The Stimson method (Fig. 2.15) was used in a minority of cases, and although this is an excellent method it is not useful in some cases because of associated injuries such as ipsilateral fractures of the femur or tibia. In this procedure the patient is placed prone on a table with the affected lower extremity hanging over the edge. Gentle pressure on the flexed knee with rotary movement will frequently effect reduction. Rough and jerky movements should be avoided. A general anesthesia gives better relaxation. However, this method has an advantage of being successful at times without a general anesthetic if that is contraindicated.

There was only one dislocation reduced after 24 hours with a good result (Table 2.3). No excellent or good results were obtained in adults reduced closed after 48 hours. The experience with adult type I dislocations in this series is similar to previous presentations of Thompson and Epstein,[100] Stewart and Milford,[95] and Brav:[9] good results occurred only in early reductions of uncomplicated dislocations. Delay in reduction in one case was caused by lack of recognition, and in another case by lack of success in an initial attempt at reduction because of the patient's poor condition. Garrett *et al.*,[34] in a recent survey of posterior dislocations, found no good results if closed reduction was performed 72 hours after surgery.

The majority of patients with type I dislocations with excellent or good results walked by the end of the 2nd month. One-third were weight-bearing by the end of the 1st month after injury (Table 2.4). There is no evidence that the time when weight-bearing was begun determined the outcome. Patients with longer periods of protection from weight-bearing did not show an increased proportion of better results. I believe that a patient should be kept in traction at about midposition of flexion of the hip for a time sufficient to heal a torn capsule—approximately 3 to 4 weeks; after traction, weight-bearing can be started with the aid of crutches. As soon as pain and muscle spasm disappear the patient may increase weight-bearing until he can eliminate the crutches.

Associated injuries (see Multiple Injuries, Chapter 8) were sustained in 28 patients with type I dislocations. Results were excellent or good in 16 and fair or poor in 12. In seven dislocations there was an ipsilateral fracture of the femur with the dislocation recognized in six and failure of recognition in one. There were five good results. In one case with a poor result the fracture was irreducible. Because of severe liver injury, open reduction was delayed for 2½ months (Fig. 2.8*A–C*).

The prompt recognition of dislocations and treatment of most patients, considering the high incidence of serious associated injuries, must be credited to the resident staff. It is our policy at Los Angeles County-University of Southern California Medical Center to take roentgenograms of the pelvis on all accident cases, including lateral and oblique views of the pelvis.

There were 20 cases of avascular necrosis in the type I dislocations (15%) (Figs. 2.7*A–D*; 2.11*A*, *B*; 2.16*A*, *B*; 2.17*A*, *B*). Seventeen had changes attributed to moderate or severe traumatic arthritis (Figs. 2.18*A–D*; 2.19*A*, *B*; 2.20*A–C*) (13%) with three cases of myositis ossificans (Fig. 2.21*A–C*) one of which occurred in a bilateral dislocation. In the miscellaneous group, four cases were rated fair clinically with normal roentgenograms. Two hips were never reduced. One patient whose hip was irreducible closed, signed out against consent (Table 2.5).

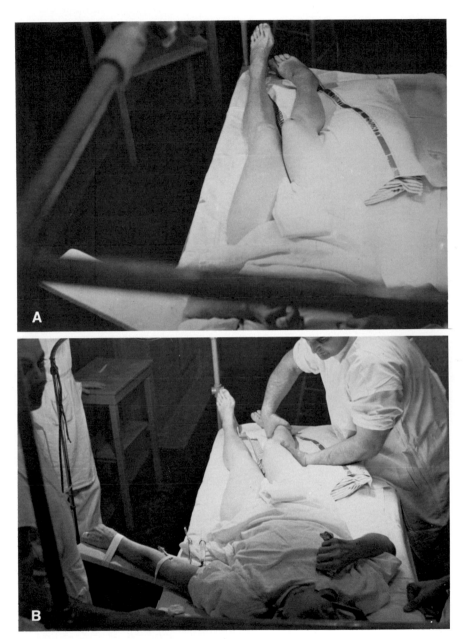

Fig. 2.14 *A,* Allis method of reduction of a posterior dislocation. *B,* traction in line of deformity.

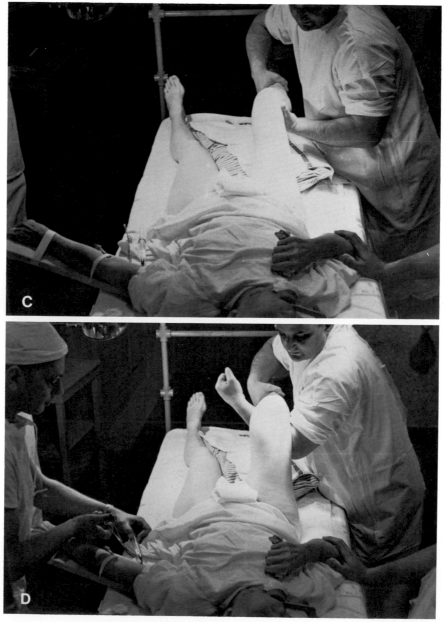

Fig. 2.14   *C*, restoration of alignment. *D*, traction with hip in flexion. (*A–C* from Epstein, H. C.: Traumatic anterior and simple posterior dislocations of the hip in adults and children. In *The American Academy of Orthopaedic Surgeons: Instructional Course Lectures,* vol. 22. The C. V. Mosby Co., St. Louis, 1973. Reproduced with permission.)

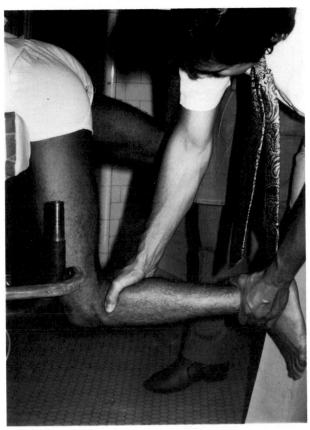

Fig. 2.15 Stimson method of reduction of a posterior dislocation of the hip. The patient is placed prone on a table with the affected leg hanging over the edge. Gentle pressure on the flexed knee with rotary movement will frequently effect reduction. Rough and jerky movements should be avoided. A general anesthesia gives better relaxation.

Table 2.3
Number of Hours before Closed Reduction Compared with Outcome in 133 Cases[a]

Number of hours before reduction									
0 to 24		25 to 48		49 or more		Not reduced		Total	
Excellent or good	Fair or poor	Excellent or good	Fair or poor	Excellent or good	Fair or poor	Excellent or good	Fair or poor	Excellent or good	Fair or poor
Number of cases									
96	24	1	1	0	7	0	3[b]	97	36

[a] Of 134 cases one was irreducible closed; opened same day with good result after long follow-up.
[b] One case reduced 2 weeks after injury; one was irreducible with open reduction 2½ months after injury; one was irreducible, the patient signed out against consent and died during subsequent surgery.

Table 2.4
Period before Full Weight-Bearing Compared with Outcome

Time in months	Excellent or good	Fair or poor
1	45	6
2	42	11
3	4	6
4	3	0
5	2	0
6	5	3
9	0	0
Unknown[a]		7
Total	101	33

[a] Outcome of seven cases: three unknown, one redislocated, two irreducible, and one never reduced.

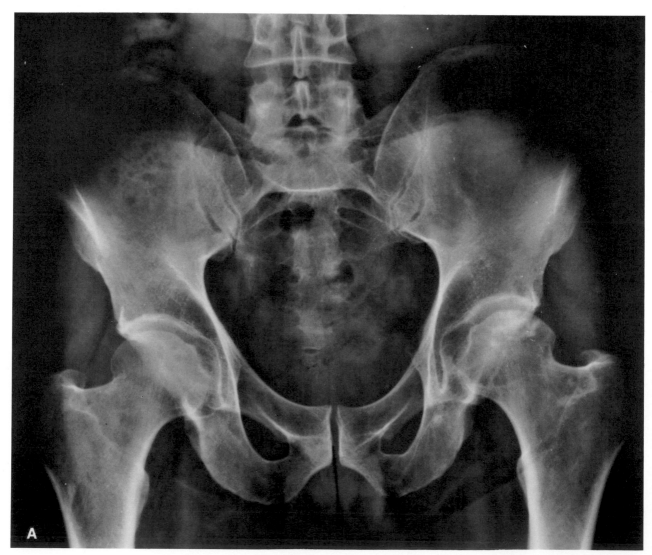

Fig. 2.16 J. I., a 34-year-old male, dislocated his left hip in an automobile vs. truck accident. The result, at 20 years, is rated good. *A*, roentgenogram made at follow-up. The original roentgenograms were lost. The hip was reduced the day of injury by the Allis method, under general anesthesia. Russell traction was maintained for 4 weeks and weight-bearing started at 8 weeks.

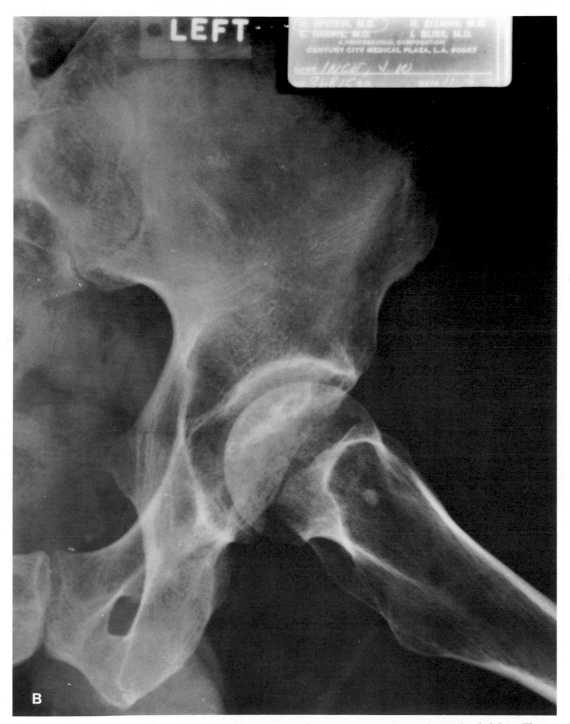

Fig. 2.16 *B,* at the last examination the patient stated he has never had any pain or discomfort in his left hip. There is, however, minimal restriction of motion. The roentgenograms indicate there could have been avascular necrosis in the early stage, since areas of increased and decreased densities are seen with some flattening of the femoral head. (*A* and *B* from Epstein, H. C.: Traumatic anterior and simple posterior dislocations of the hip in adults and children. In *The American Academy of Orthopaedic Surgeons: Instructional Course Lectures,* vol. 22. The C. V. Mosby Co., St. Louis, 1973. Reproduced with permission.)

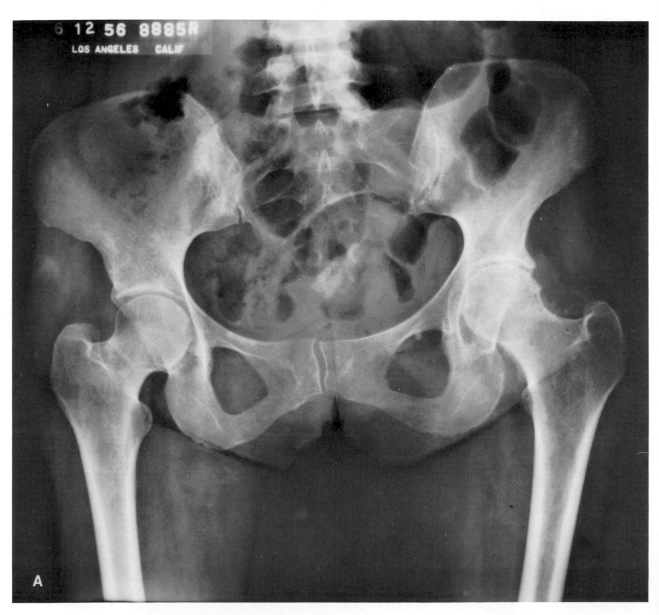

Fig. 2.17 B. P., a 32-year-old woman, dislocated her left hip when her car went over a bridge. She sustained a type I dislocation with an ipsilateral fracture of the femur (supracondylar). The patient had a compound fracture of the left tibia and a pulmonary embolus. *A,* twenty-six months later the result is rated poor with avascular necrosis. The dislocation was not recognized for 2 weeks. It was reduced by a private physician in Arizona.

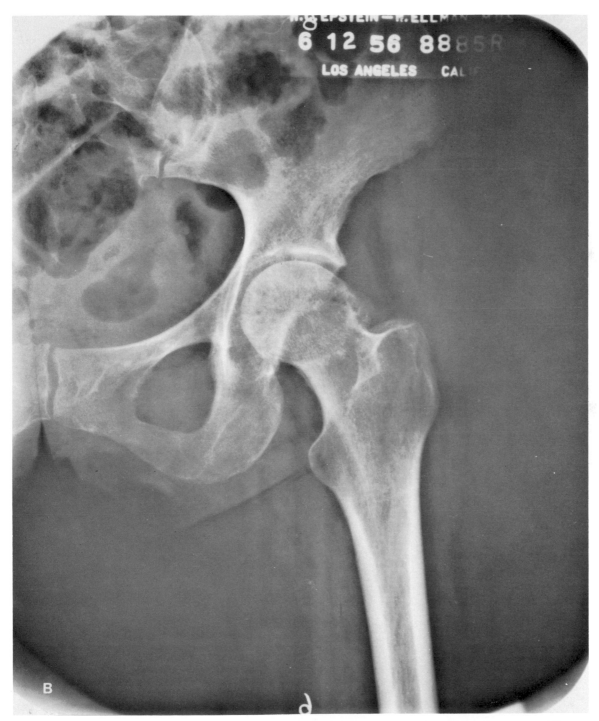

Fig. 2.17 *B,* anteroposterior and lateral roentgenograms made 26 months after injury show avascular necrosis. The patient had severe hip pain and moderate restriction of motions. Avascular necrosis was first noted 13 months after injury.

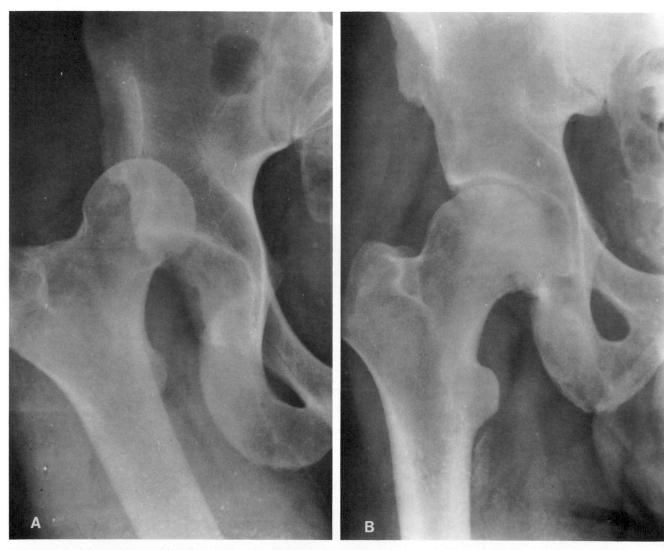

Fig. 2.18   A. M., a 36-year-old male, sustained a simple posterior dislocation, a dashboard injury in an automobile accident. The result was rated good in 4 years but poor in 13 years. *A,* the hip was reduced closed the day of injury. The patient had Russell traction for 10 days and was weight-bearing at 2 months. *B,* four years after injury the patient was examined at the author's office, with a good result.

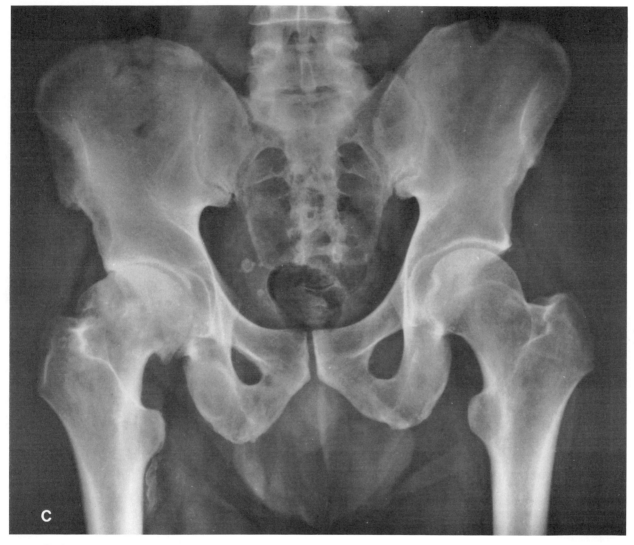

Fig. 2.18 C, thirteen years later, the patient had pain and limitation of motion of the hip. The roentgenogram reveals moderate narrowing of the hip joint with moderate spur formation, superiorly and inferiorly.

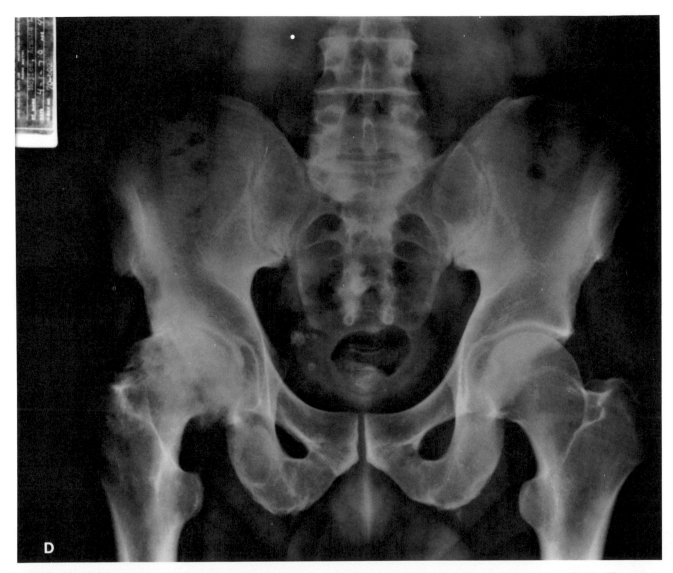

Fig. 2.18 *D*, seventeen years after injury, the roentgenogram shows more advanced changes of traumatic arthritis. The patient had more pain and was unable to get about his normal activities. He subsequently had a cup arthroplasty with satisfactory return of hip function. (*A–D* from Epstein, H. C.: Traumatic anterior and simple posterior dislocations of the hip in adults and children. In *The American Academy of Orthopaedic Surgeons: Instructional Course Lectures,* vol. 22. The C. V. Mosby Co., St. Louis, 1973. Reproduced with permission.)

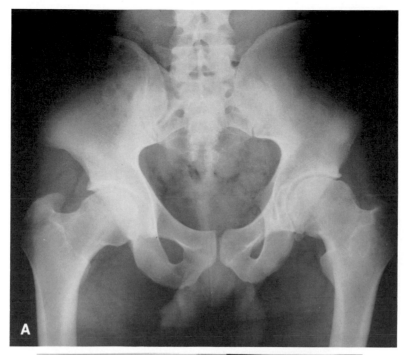

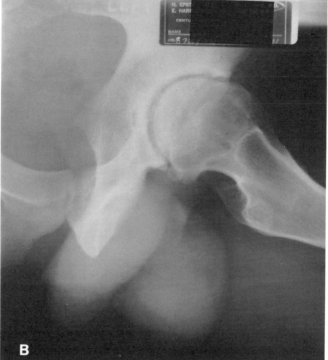

Fig. 2.19 F. H., a 22-year-old man, sustained a type I dislocation of his left hip in a motorcycle vs. automobile collision. The result, 8½ years later, is fair. *A,* the hip was reduced under general anesthesis the day of injury. Buck's traction was applied for 3 weeks and patient walked at 4 weeks. *B,* there is moderate limitation of left hip motion, with a 20° flexion contracture and limp on weight-bearing. The roentgenogram reveals moderate narrowing of the hip joint with osteophytes and some flattening of the head of the femur.

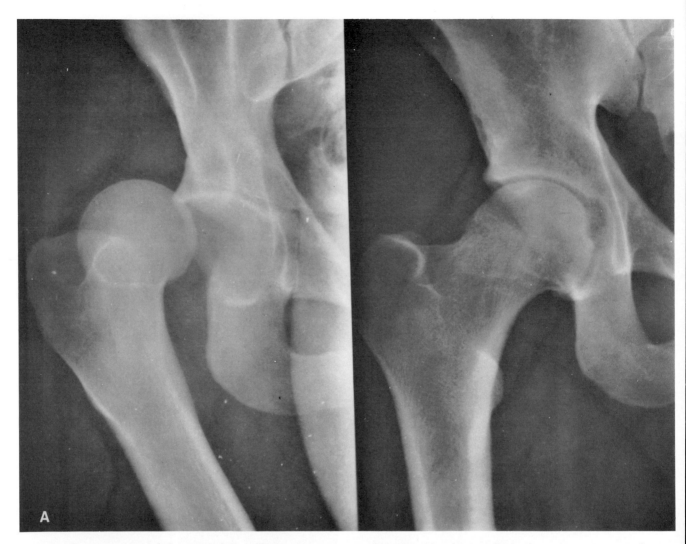

Fig. 2.20 Posterior type I dislocation of the right hip in an 18 year-old male with a fair result. *A,* the patient was injured in an automobile vs. pole accident. The hip was reduced, closed, under general anesthesia the day of injury. Buck's traction was maintained for 3 weeks and full weight-bearing was started the 4th week.

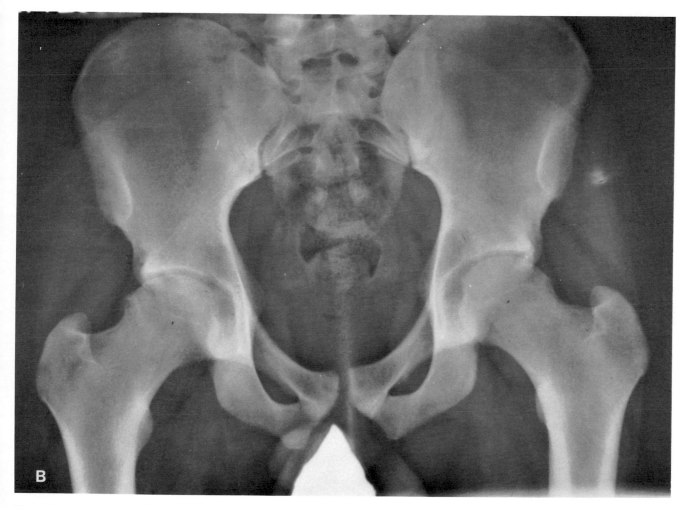

Fig. 2.20   *B,* at 3½ years later there is minimal narrowing of the hip joint. The patient has pain and discomfort in the hip.

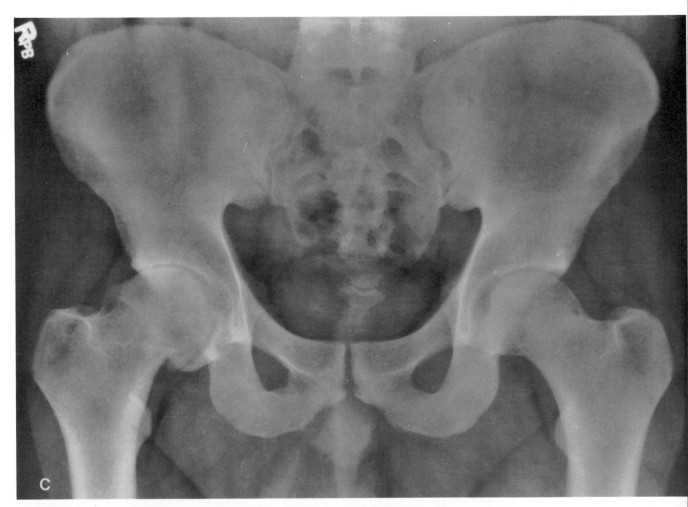

Fig. 2.20   C, at 5½ years after injury there is more narrowing of the hip joint, with osteophytes at the junction of the head and neck superiorly and inferiorly. The patient has moderate limitation of hip motion and pain.

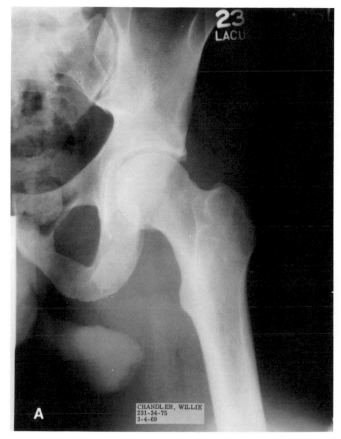

Fig. 2.21 W. C., a 35-year-old male, sustained a posterior type I dislocation of the left hip in an auto accident. At the time of the accident the patient also sustained an acute thoracic trauma. The result of his dislocation, 20 months later, was fair with moderate myositis ossificans. *A,* reduction performed under local 1% Xylocaine into the hip joint, because of the chest injury. The patient refused to allow Russell traction and after discharge at 4 weeks he started weight-bearing.

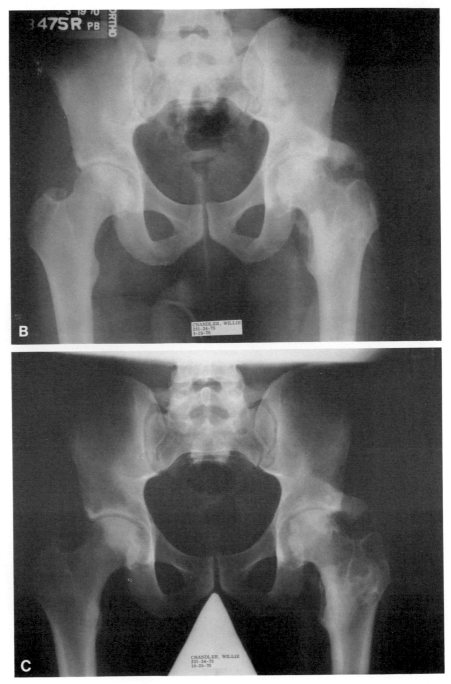

Fig. 2.21 *B,* one year later there is myositis ossificans around the left hip joint. *C,* twenty months after injury the myositis ossificans is more pronounced. There is moderate restriction of hip motion, with pain and aching in the hip.

Table 2.5
Incidence of Roentgenographic Joint Changes in 47 Fair or Poor Results in Type I Dislocations in Adults[a]

	Avascular necrosis	Traumatic arthritis	Myositis ossificans	Miscellaneous	Fair or poor
Total	20	17	3	7[a]	47
Percentage	15	13	2	5	

[a] Four hips fair clinically, x-rays normal; two hips never reduced; one hip irreducible (patient signed out and died in surgery 3 months later).

Amstrong[3] reported that traumatic arthritis occurred in 15% of patients with dislocations without a fracture. Stewart and Milford[95] reported that in a total of 25 type I dislocations, avascular necrosis appeared in three cases (12%). Brav[9] reported 24 cases of avascular necrosis (22%) and 29 cases with traumatic arthritis (26%) in a total of 110 type I dislocations.

DISTRIBUTION AND NERVE INJURIES

There were 18 nerve injuries in type I dislocations in adults, 8 sciatic and 10 peroneal. These will be discussed in Chapter 11, Nerve Injuries.

RECURRENT DISLOCATIONS OF THE HIP

Three patients had clinical and roentgenographic evidence of recurrent dislocations of the same hip. One had three separate incidents resulting in dislocations over a 5-year period. The result after the last dislocation was poor (Fig. 2.22A–F). One patient with a long follow-up dislocated the same hip in an automobile accident on two separate occasions 16 years apart. The result 22 years later was good (Fig. 2.23A, B). The third patient dislocated the same hip in two minor incidents approximately 1 year apart; both times the patient fell down the stairs. On follow-up after each accident the result was good (Fig. 2.24A–D). Two patients gave presumptive evidence of having dislocated the same hip on numerous occasions, but no record was available to confirm or deny their histories. One had a poor result and one had a good result. None of the patients with recurrent dislocations had undergone open reduction for the repeated dislocations, according to Wilson[112] and Rowe and Lowell.[89]

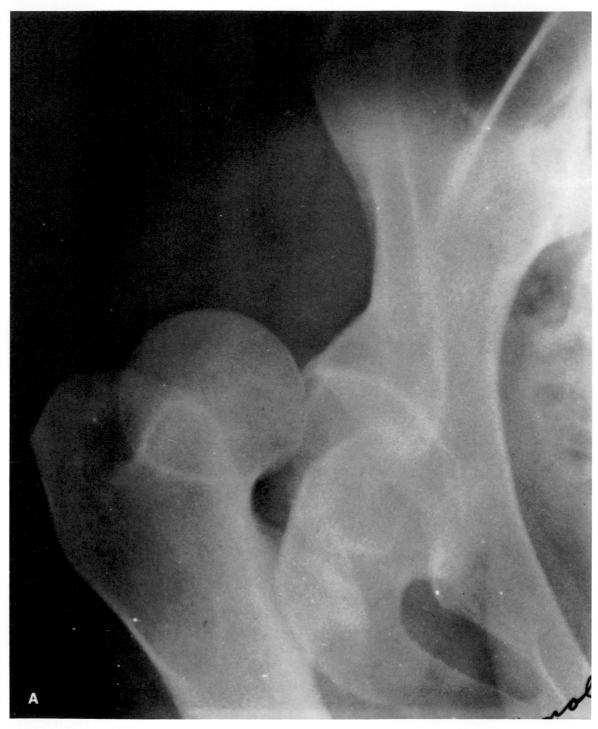

Fig. 2.22 McK., a female, sustained posterior dislocations on three separate occasions, in the same hip, over a 5-year period. On April 19, 1932, this 29-year-old woman dislocated her right hip when she jumped out of a second story window. Reduction was accomplished within 20 hours after injury; she was maintained in traction for 6 weeks and discharged. She was seen in the Trauma Clinic 4 months later without complaints. *A*, this is a simple type I dislocation without fracture.

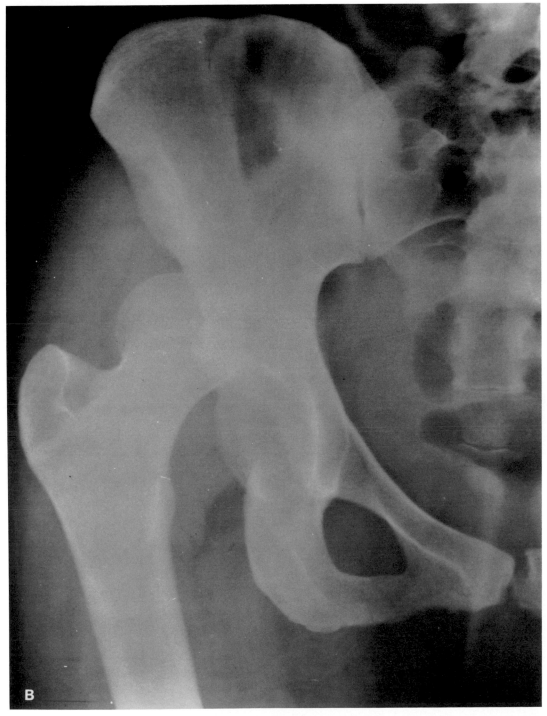

Fig. 2.22 *B,* on September 23, 1936, the same hip was dislocated when the patient was involved in an automobile accident. It was reduced the same day. Weight-bearing was started 1 month later.

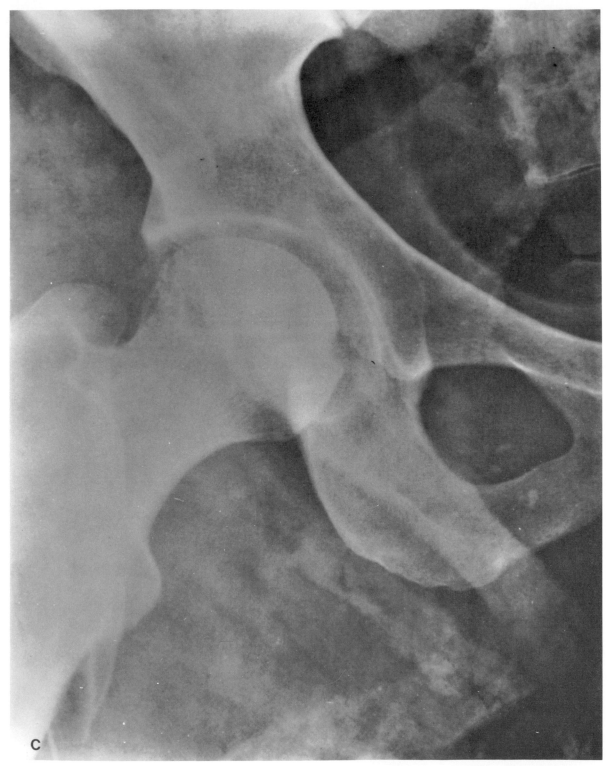

Fig. 2.22 *C,* roentgenogram made on September 25, 1936, shows reduction of the second dislocation. Note the myositis ossificans of the lesser trochanter.

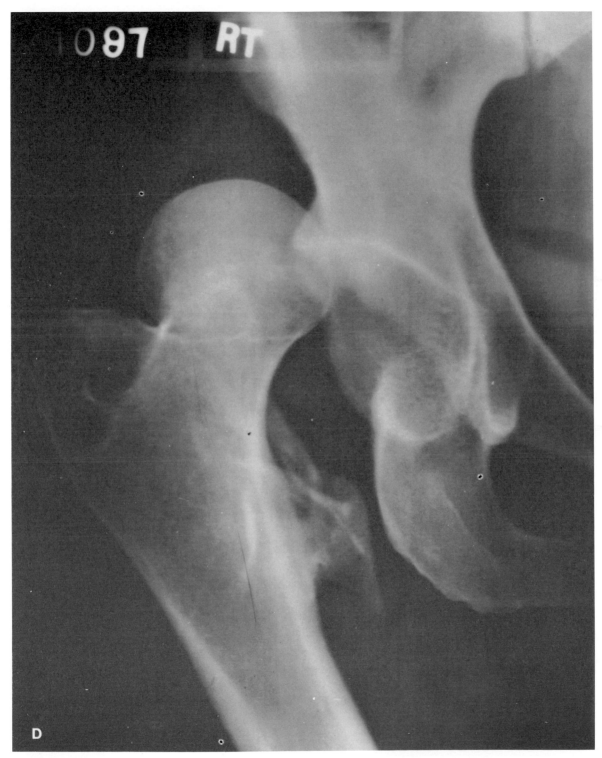

Fig. 2.22 *D,* on August 20, 1937, the patient was thrown out of an automobile. Again, the same hip was dislocated. Note the extra bone over the lesser trochanter.

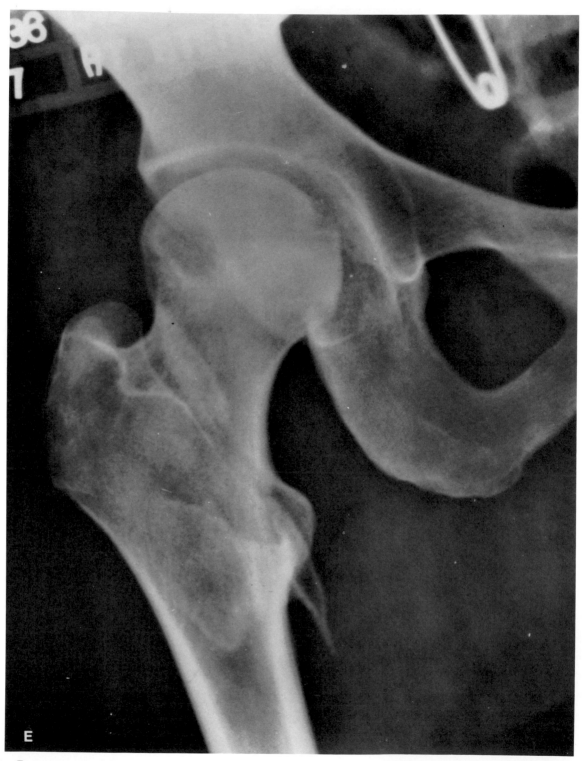

Fig. 2.22 *E,* an unsuccessful attempt at reduction of the hip was made on August 24, 1937. It was successfully reduced on September 3, 1937, and a spica cast was applied. The patient was followed in the clinic for 1 month.

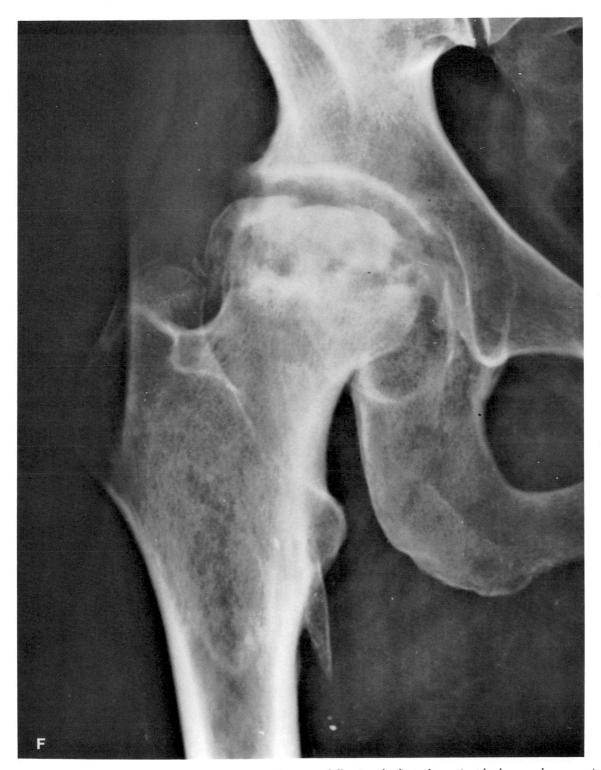

F

Fig. 2.22 *F,* three years following the last dislocation, and 8 years following the first, the patient had avascular necrosis of the femoral head. (*A–F* from Epstein, H. C.: Traumatic anterior and simple posterior dislocations of the hip in adults and children. In *The American Academy of Orthopaedic Surgeons: Instructional Course Lectures,* vol. 22. The C. V. Mosby Co., St. Louis, 1973. Reproduced with permission.)

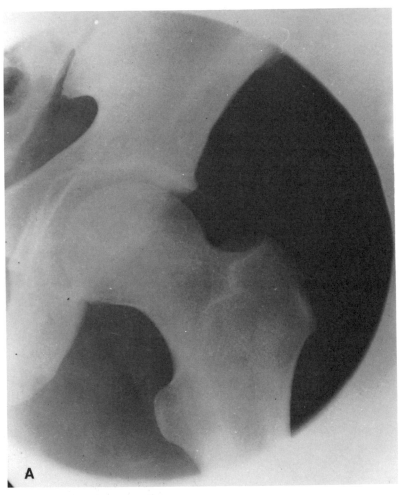

Fig. 2.23   A 17-year-old male dislocated his left hip in an automobile vs. tree accident (type I) in September 1948. It was reduced under general anesthesia by the Allis method, 48 hours after injury. The patient was maintained in Russell traction for 1 week and a spica cast for 5 months, and then weight-bearing with a good result 2 years after injury. *A,* at 16 years and 3 months later, at age 33, the patient dislocated the same left hip in an automobile vs. truck accident. The hip was reduced the day of injury, under iv morphine sulfate, by the Stimson maneuver. He was placed in Buck's traction for 3 weeks and started weight-bearing in 4 weeks.

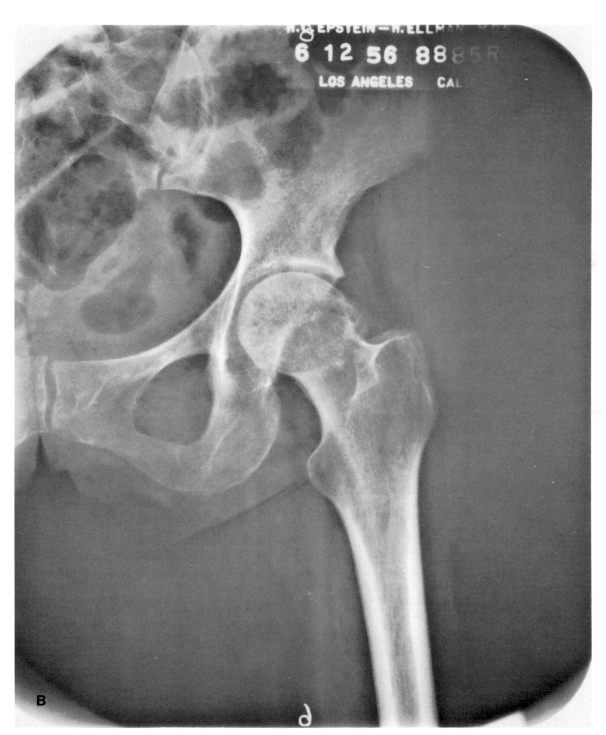

Fig. 2.23 *B,* the result, 22 years and 8 months later, is good. There is minimal restriction of hip motion without complaints.

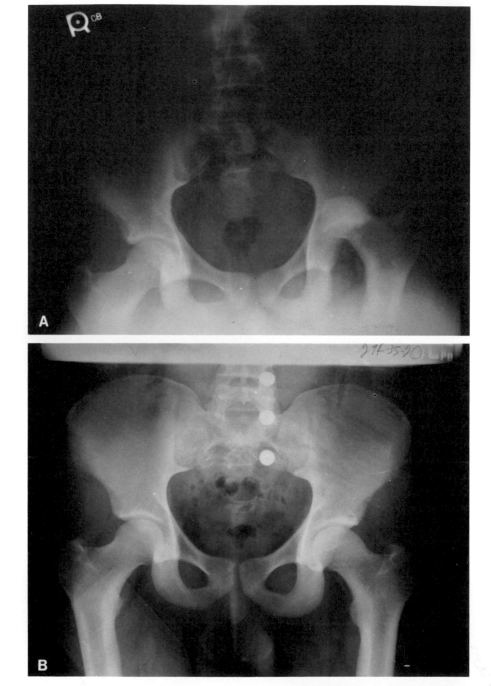

Fig. 2.24   A. Z., a 17-year-old male, sustained posterior dislocation of the left hip on two separate occasions. *A,* on February 8, 1969, he slipped and fell down two flights of stairs, dislocating the left hip. *B,* the hip was reduced under general anesthesia by the Allis method, the same day. He was in traction 6 weeks and weight-bearing at 7 weeks, with an excellent result at 12 months.

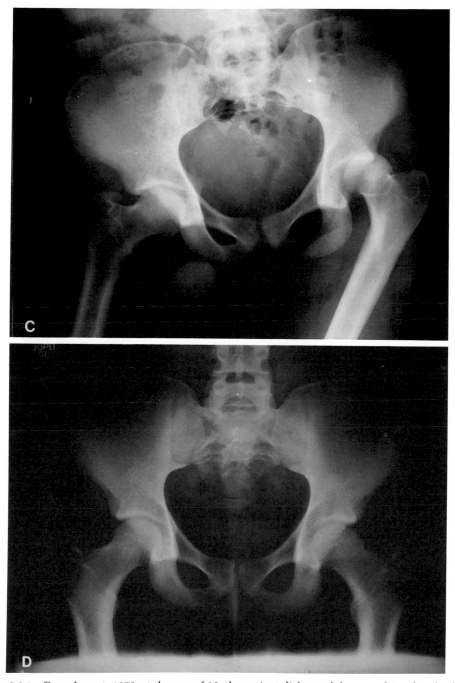

Fig. 2.24 *C*, on June 6, 1970, at the age of 18, the patient dislocated the same hip when he fell down some stairs. He was in traction 6 weeks and then started weight-bearing. *D*, roentgenogram made in February, 1971. There is minimal limitation of hip motion and minimal narrowing of the hip joint although the result, so far is considered good.

CHAPTER
3

FRACTURE-DISLOCATIONS

In a study of 204 traumatic dislocations of the hip completed in 1950, Thompson and Epstein[100] found that the results were satisfactory only in anterior and simple posterior type I dislocations.

The unsatisfactory results in the posterior fracture-dislocations occurred when open reduction was delayed or when closed methods were used in the presence of small loose fragments within the joint space. In 1958, in a study of 55 cases of posterior fracture-dislocations,[27] the results of open reduction of the hip were compared with those obtained by closed methods. The open procedures were performed to remove loose fragments from the joint space, to restore stability to the joint by open reduction and internal fixation of any large fragments of the posterior rim of the acetabulum, and to ensure accurate reduction of the dislocation. The findings in this study revealed that for fracture-dislocations of the hip, primary open reduction gave results superior to those obtained by closed reduction followed by an open procedure and also superior to those obtained by closed reduction alone.

Urist,[104] in 1948, recommended primary open reduction of dislocations associated with comminuted fractures of the acetabulum. Stewart and Milford[95] and Brav[9] advised open procedures only when closed reduction failed, when loose fragments were visible in the joint on roentgenograms, or when the joint was unstable. Gordon and Freiberg[38] recommended excision of the head fragment in a fracture dislocation which involved the femoral head. King and Richards[60] demonstrated that, apparently because of incongruity of the joint surfaces, rapid disintegration occurred in the hip joints of dogs when reduction of the fracture-dislocation was incomplete.

After a long-term follow-up of 242 posterior fracture-dislocations of the hip printed in *The Journal of Bone and Joint Surgery*, September 1974,[25] it was again concluded that early primary open reductions offered the best prognosis. By definition, *primary open reduction* means that closed reduction is not attempted and that fragments of bone and cartilage, some of which are not visible on roentgenograms, are removed surgically before reduction. That such fragments are frequently present is substantiated by this study. Only 11 of the 176 open procedures (closed reduction followed by open reduction and primary open reduction) specifically failed to demonstrate fragments in the hip joint, while the operative note for eight others failed to mention whether fragments were found or not, although the joint spaces were irrigated. The sizes of the fragments in the remaining hips ranged from small ones not visible on the roentgenogram to some that were 0.25 cm in diameter. Bony fragments or debris were found in the hip joint at surgery in 91% of the cases.

RESULTS

The results were rated according to the type of lesion in the 116 hips treated by closed reduction, in the 93 treated by closed followed by open procedures and in the 83 treated by primary open reduction. The results in the three groups were then compared.

CLOSED REDUCTION

Of the 116 hips treated by closed reduction, 22 were type II, 42 were type III, 38 were type IV, and 17 were type V (Table 3.1).

Type II

In the 22 type II hips (in 22 patients) (Fig. 3.1A, B), there were seven good (Fig. 3.2A–C), seven fair, and eight poor results. Eight of the 15 patients with fair or poor results had had unfavorable features. These included delay of reduction until 3 and 9 days after injury in two; no reduction in four (hip injury not recognized at all during treatment on one, not recognized for 9 days because of an ipsilteral fracture of the femoral shaft in another, not recognized for 1 month in the third, and recognized but no reduction attempted in the fourth because of the patient's poor general condition); and two redislocations 1 month and 3 months after reduction. Of the remaining seven patients with unsatisfactory results, one had an anterior dislocation on one side and a posterior fracture dislocation on the other, both reduced on the day of injury with subsequent marked myositis ossificans about both hips (Fig. 3.3). Another had three attempts at reduction over a 5-day interval before reduction was accomplished (Fig. 1.32*A–C*), while the other five had dislocations that were reduced on the day of injury on the first attempt with no instability of the hip following reduction.

Table 3.1
Results in 116 Posterior Fracture-Dislocations According to Type: Closed Reductions

Type	Good	Fair	Poor	Total	Percentage of good results
II	7	7	8	22	32
III	1	16	25	42	20
IV	5	10	23	38	13
V	0	6	8	14	0
Total	13	39	64	116	12

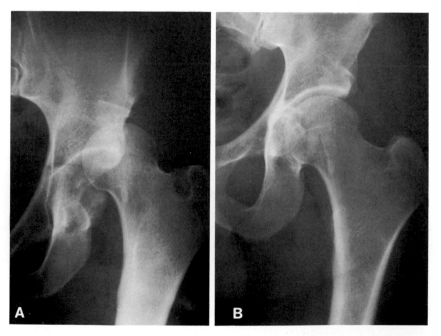

Fig. 3.1   A 31-year-old male involved in an auto accident as a passenger. Type II closed reduction was performed. Follow-up at 29 months showed good result. Patient had sustained fracture-dislocation of left hip, cerebral concussion, compound fracture right maxilla, fracture of right humerus and wrist, and fracture of left femur. *A,* roentgenogram July 24, 1955, closed reduction on day of injury. Patient was in traction 2 months; hip spica for fractured femur, 6 months; full weight-bearing at the end of 8 months. *B,* roentgenogram October 30, 1957. Joint space is normal. There is no traumatic arthritis and no avascular necrosis. Posterior acetabular rim fragment was not repositioned anatomically. Range of hip motion is good, without pain. Patient is able to work normally.

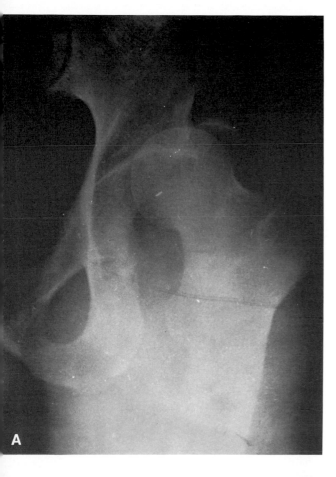

Fig. 3.2 A 52-year-old man in an auto vs. truck accident was thrown out of the car and dislocated his left hip. This is a type II injury with a large fragment off the posterior acetabular rim. A closed reduction was accomplished under a general anesthetic on the day of injury; a peroneal palsy returned to normal by the 4th month. The result after 9 years and 1 month was good. *A,* roentgenogram reveals posterior dislocation with a large posterior rim fragment displaced superiorly. *B,* after a closed reduction. The joint space appears normal. Traction was used for 1 month, then a spica cast for 6 weeks, followed by weight-bearing. *C,* at follow-up there is no narrowing of hip joint and no avascular necrosis. The fractured acetabular rim is not anatomically repositioned. There is no hip pain and no limping but patient has mild discomfort in hip after a day's work.

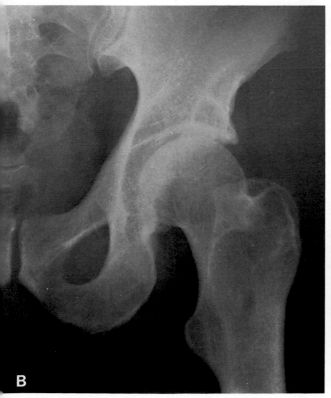

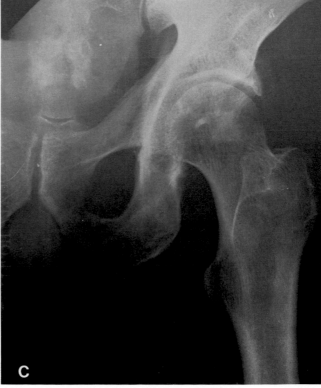

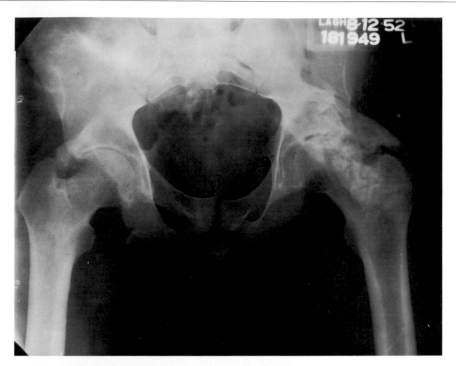

Fig. 3.3 This 43-year-old patient sustained a bilateral dislocation, posterior type II on right and obturator on the left, when involved in an auto accident. Both hips were reduced under general anesthesia, method unknown. He was transferred to the Los Angeles County Hospital 3 weeks later. Roentgenograms revealed reduction of both hips although there appeared to be a small portion of bone avulsed off the posterior acetabular rim on the left side. One month after injury calcification was noted superiorly over both hips. At 49 months after injury there was moderate myositis ossificans with almost complete bony bridging over left hip. The patient walked with marked lumbar lordosis but no definite hip pain. Patient also had a frozen right shoulder and calcification about his right elbow. The result of the dislocated hips was fair.

In this study, *not reduced* implies that the head of the femur was not in its normal relationship to the acetabululm. In all seven hips with good results the dislocation was reduced within 24 hours on the first attempt and the reduced hip appeared to be stable even though the posterior acetabular rim fragment remained displaced posteriorly after reduction.

Type III

In the 42 type III hips (in 42 patients) there was one good result (after a follow-up of 8 1/2 years), 16 fair, and 25 poor results. The good result was in a 40-year-old man who had his dislocation reduced on the day of injury by the Allis method and had Russell traction applied for 1 month. He then walked with a cane for 2 months, resuming full weight-bearing 3 months after injury. At follow-up his only discomfort was noted while getting up from a sitting position; he also had a feeling of stiffness in cold weather but no pain. Roentgenograms showed no evidence of traumatic arthritis or avascular necrosis (Fig. 3.4A–C).

Of the 41 patients with unsatisfactory results, two had had no attempt at reduction because of their poor condition; one fell and fractured his hip 2 months after reduction, with a subsequent poor result; two, because the diagnosis was missed, had delayed reductions, 48 hours and 6 weeks after injury, with fair and poor results, respectively; one, whose primary open reduction was canceled

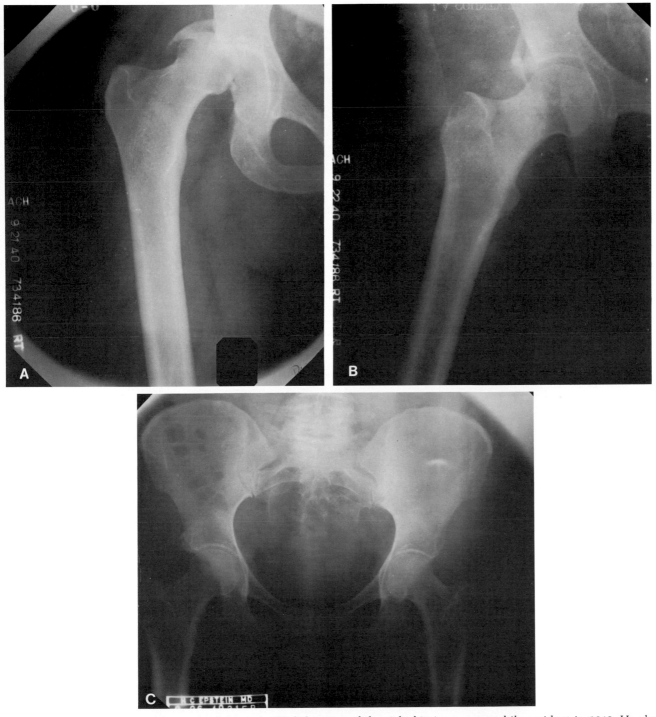

Fig. 3.4 A male, 40 years old, sustained this type III dislocation of the right hip in an automobile accident in 1940. He also sustained an ipsilateral lateral tibial plateau fracture. The result 9½ years after a closed reduction was rated good. *A*, roentgenogram made on the day of injury. Note the comminuted fragments about the hip joint. *B*, roentgenogram after a closed reduction performed under general anesthesia on the day of injury. Russell traction was used for 28 days. Patient used a cane for 2 months. There was no difficulty with the hip after 3 months. *C*, roentgenogram made at follow-up. There was minimal limitation of internal rotation of the hip. The patient works as an electrician, which involves considerable ladder climbing. There is no discomfort after sitting and there is no pain.

because of furuncles in the buttock on the involved side, had a poor result after closed reduction; one was admitted with his hip still dislocated 15 months after injury; one, whose hip was unstable after reduction, refused an open procedure; two had multiple attempts before reduction was accomplished; one, after closed reduction, refused open reduction to remove fragments from the hip joint; eight, whose hip joint was wide or who had fragments roentgenographically visible in the hip joint after reduction, did not have open reduction, and 22 had closed reduction on the day of injury on the first attempt, one of them being a child. (Figs. 3.5A–C; 3.6A–C; 3.7A–C).

It is probable that many of these 41 unfavorable results could have been prevented. Thompson and Epstein[100] stated that there are good reasons to believe that the results in type III hips may be improved by removing the loose fragments in the joint, since these appear to be one cause of unfavorable results. Failure to recognize a dislocation or to reduce a dislocation successfully on the first attempt within 24 hours after injury also contributes to unsatisfactory results.

Type IV

In the 38 type IV hips (in 38 patients) there were five good, 10 fair, and 23 poor results (Figs. 3.8A–C; 3.9A–C; 3.10A–D; 3.11A–C; 3.12A–E). Of the five good results, four were in patients in whom the superior weight-bearing dome of the acetabulum was not involved and whose dislocations were reduced on the day of

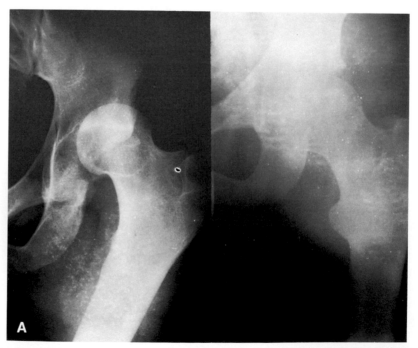

Fig. 3.5 A man, 22 years old, in an automobile accident sustained a posterior dislocation of the left hip with a comminuted but not grossly displaced acetabular fracture. At follow-up, 6 months later, the patient had traumatic arthritis and the result was rated poor. A, roentgenogram made on day of injury reveals a type III dislocation. On the first attempt at reduction the femoral head slipped anteriorly. It was pushed back posteriorly and then reduced into the acetabulum. Check roentgenograms of the reduction was accepted although the films were very light.

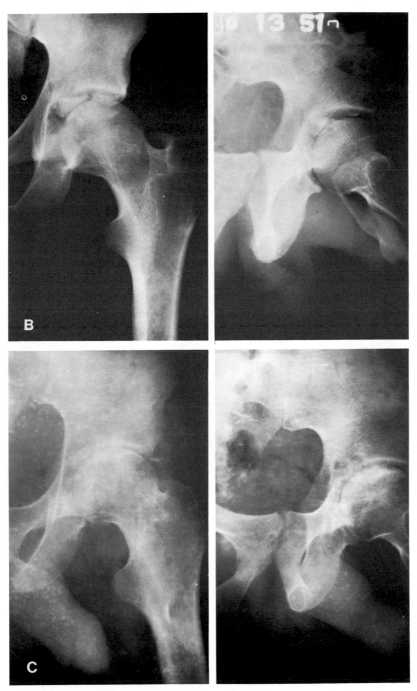

Fig. 3.5 *B,* anterior-posterior and lateral roentgenograms made 1 month after reduction reveal widening of the joint space with loose fragments within the joint. No attempt was made to remove the fragments. *C,* anterior-posterior and lateral roentgenograms made 6 months after injury revealed moderate narrowing of the joint space with increased sclerosis about the acetabulum and femoral head, which shows mottling. The lateral view shows irregularity and depression of the weight-bearing portion of the head. The patient has moderate limitation of motion of the hip with pain.

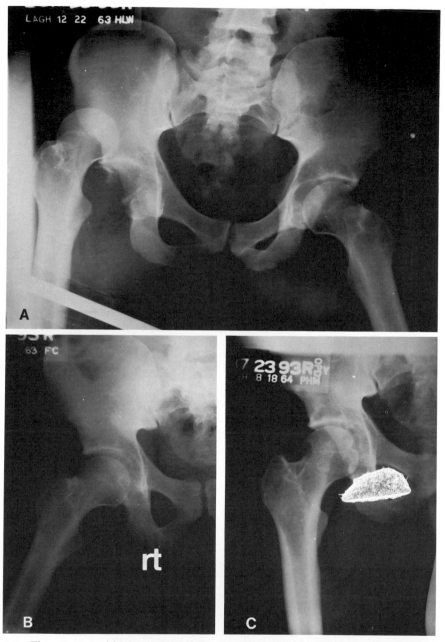

Fig. 3.6 This 27-year-old man sustained this type III posterior dislocation when struck by an automobile. Numerous attempts at closed reduction were unsuccesful by the Allis method of reduction under a general anesthesia. The patient was then intubated and reduction was accomplished by the Stimson method. Nine months after reduction there is traumatic arthritis and the result is fair. *A,* roentgenogram on day of injury. Note the numerous small fragments of bone about the hip joint. *B,* roentgenogram after reduction. The joint space was wider than the opposite hip with evidence of loose fragments within the joint. *C,* at last follow-up there is traumatic arthritis with a bony fragment within the joint. The patient has distress in his hip with long periods of ambulation.

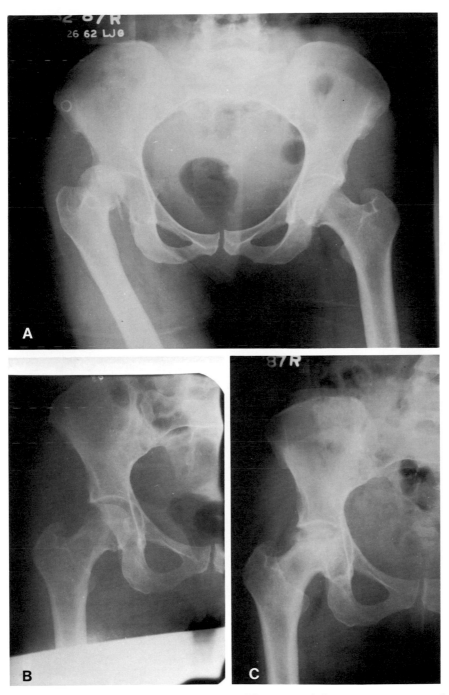

Fig. 3.7 A 45-year-old woman sustained this type III posterior dislocation in an auto accident. There were multiple injuries including fractured ribs, a fracture of the mandible, and a ruptured spleen. A closed reduction was accomplished prior to abdominal surgery. The patient was kept in traction for 26 days and started weight-bearing 3 months later. The result, 38 months after injury, was poor with avascular necrosis. *A*, roentgenogram reveals posterior dislocation with multiple loose fragments within the joint. *B*, roentgenogram after reduction reveals a wide joint space (compared to opposite hip) with a fragment of bone within the superior portion of the hip joint. *C*, roentgenogram at follow-up reveals avascular necrosis with irregularity and flattening of the femoral head. The patient did well until 3 years after injury, when she slowly developed hip pain which is, now, constant.

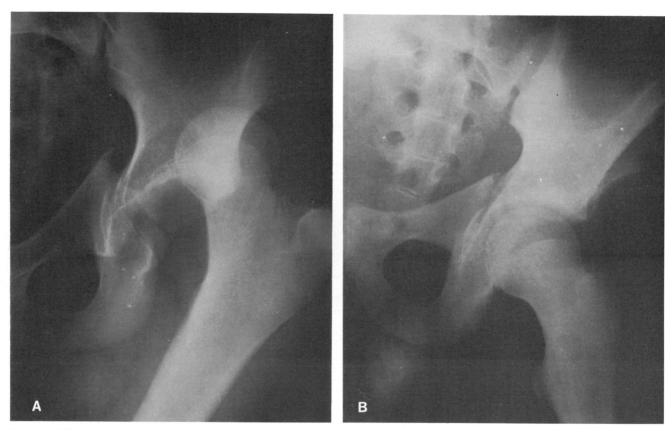

Fig. 3.8   This 17-year-old man was injured in a collision of two trucks, sustaining this type IV posterior dislocation of the right hip. A closed reduction was performed on the day of injury and the result 12 years and 9 months later was rated good. *A*, roentgenogram taken on day of injury reveals a large fragment of the posterior superior rim of the acetabulum with the fracture of the floor of the acetabulum occurring through the triradiate cartilage, *B*, after reduction the hip resembles a central protrusion fracture. The dome of the acetabulum is not involved. The large fracture of the posterior acetabular rim is displaced superiorly.

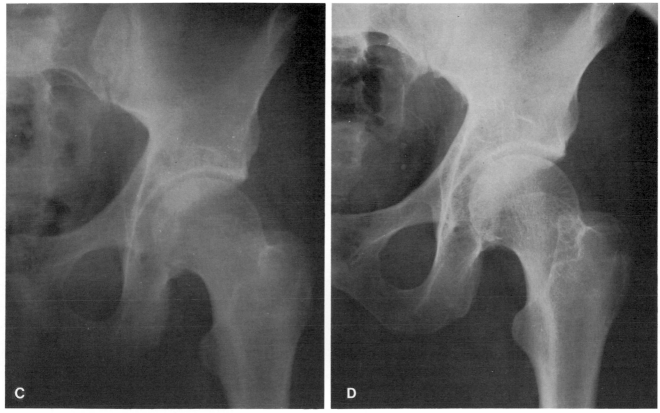

Fig. 3.8 *C*, roentgenogram made 4 years later. The patient had some stiffness but no pain, although pain had persisted for 3 years. Full weight-bearing had been resumed 3 months after the injury. *D*, roentgenogram made 12 years and 9 months later. There was no pain but the patient had some discomfort after dancing or hard work. Note the change in the trabecular pattern of the head and the slight irregularity of the subchondral cortex.

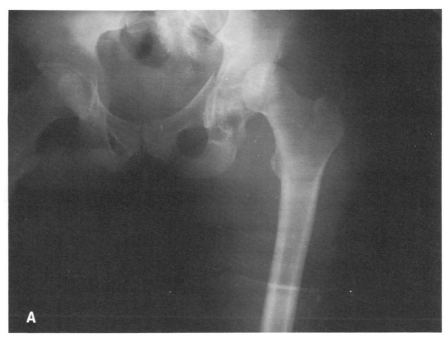

Fig. 3.9 This 26-year-old male sustained a type IV posterior dislocation of the left hip plus an ipsilateral traumatic amputation above the knee in a motorcycle vs. automobile accident. The dislocation of the hip was not recognized for 2 days. A closed reduction was performed. The result 45 months later is fair with moderate myositis ossificans. *A*, roentgenogram taken 2 days after injury. There is a posterior dislocation with comminuted fractures through the floor of the acetabulum.

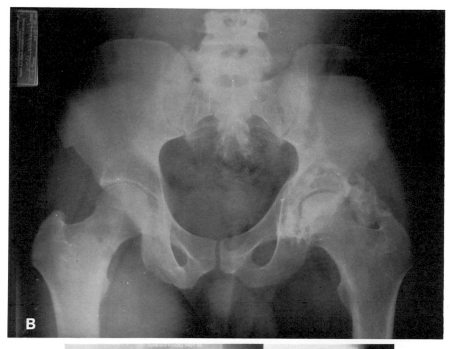

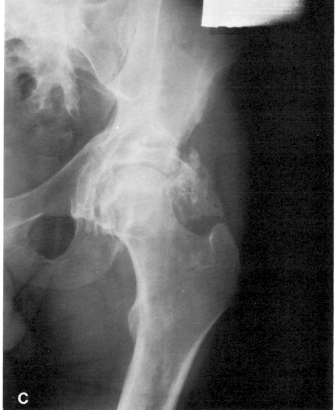

Fig. 3.9 *B,* roentgenogram taken 6 months after reduction reveals heterotopic bone formation. *C,* roentgenogram at check-up 45 months after injury. There is a mature myositis ossificans with minimal narrowing of the joint space. Patient complained of constant aching pain in his hip.

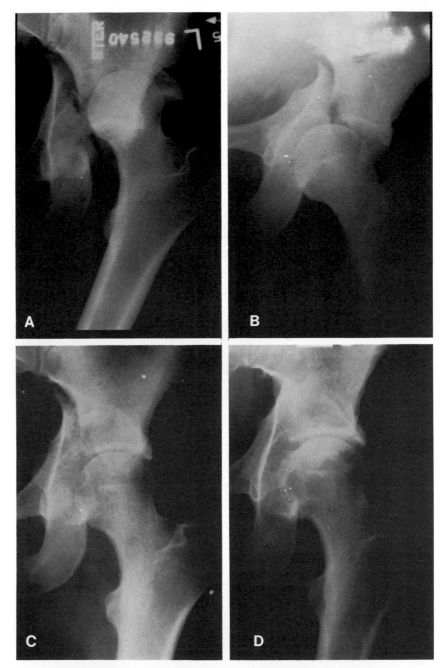

Fig. 3.10   A 19-year-old woman sustained this type IV posterior dislocation in an automobile accident. A closed reduction was done on the day of injury under spinal anesthesia. The result 58 months later was rated fair with traumatic arthritis. A, roentgenogram on day of injury. There is a large fragment involving the posterior superior acetabular rim plus a comminuted fracture through the floor of the acetabulum. B, after reduction the dislocation resembles a central protrusion fracture with medial migration of the femoral head. The dome of the acetabulum is involved. C, roentgenogram 4 months after reduction. The posterior column fracture is uniting with minimum narrowing of the joint space. D, roentgenogram at follow-up. There has been complete healing of the acetabular fracture with minimal narrowing of the hip joint. There are scattered areas of increased densities in the femoral head. The patient has no pain and is able to walk one mile without hip pain; also had recent pregnancy. She was rated fair because of roentgenographic findings.

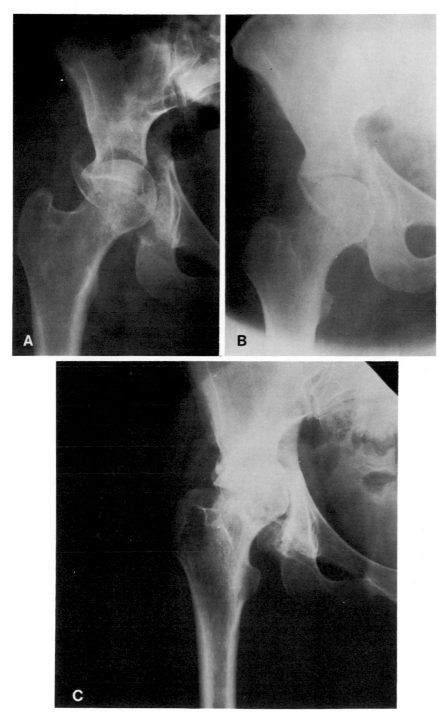

Fig. 3.11 A 46-year-old woman sustained this type IV posterior dislocation in an automobile accident. She was admitted to the LAC/USC Medical Center 13 days later. A closed reduction was performed. The result 17 months later was rated poor with traumatic arthritis. *A,* roentgenogram on day of admission. There is a fracture through the floor and roof of the acetabulum involving the weight-bearing portion of the dome. *B,* roentgenogram on day of admission. There is a fracture through the floor and roof of the acetabulum involving the weight-bearing portion of the dome. *B,* roentgenogram taken after closed reduction. There is medial displacement of the femoral head. The posterior-superior acetabular rim fragment is not anatomically repositioned. *C,* roentgenogram at last visit. There is complete obliteration of the joint space with areas of increased and decreased densities throughout the femoral head. The patient had considerable pain with marked restriction of motion of the hip.

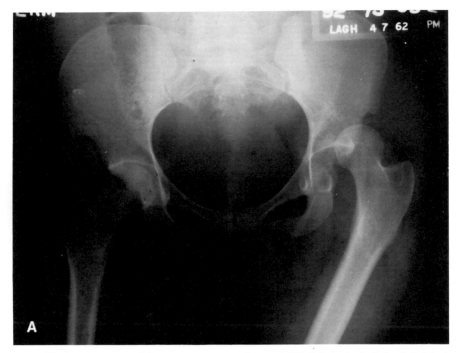

Fig. 3.12 V. A., a 23-year-old woman, sustained a type IV dislocation of the left hip in an auto accident on April 7, 1962. The result 4 years after closed reduction was rated poor with avascular necrosis. A, roentgenogram taken at the time of injury reveals a fragment off the superior rim of the acetabulum. It is difficult to visualize the fracture through the floor of the acetabulum.

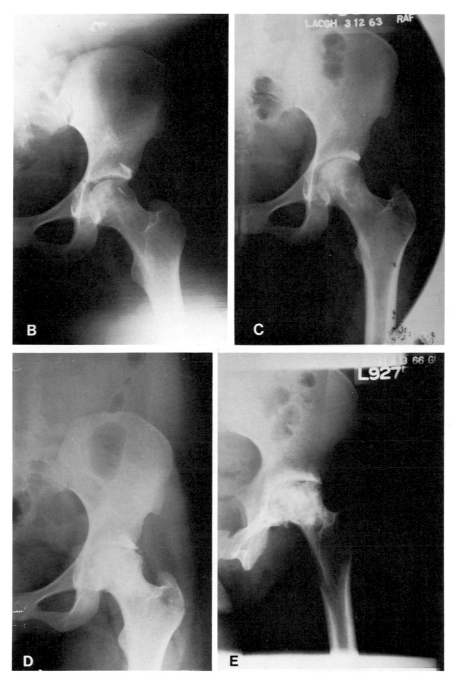

Fig. 3.12 *B,* reduction roentgenogram taken on the day of injury, after a closed reduction, 26 hours postinjury. Traction was maintained for 6 weeks and weight-bearing started at 4 months. *C,* Eleven months after injury, roentgenogram reveals no evidence of avascular necrosis. Patient started having pain in the left hip ten months after injury. *D,* three years after injury there are now definite changes in the femoral head with flattening of the femoral head at the superior weight-bearing portion and areas of increased and decreased densities throughout the femoral head. Patient was having severe pain with marked limitation of motion. *E,* roentgenogram reveals more advanced changes of avascular necrosis in the femoral head. There is now collapse of the weight-bearing portion, with more pronounced areas of increased densities. The joint space appears to be well maintained.

the injury. The remaining good result was in a man last seen 12 years after injury, which had occurred when he was 17 years old. The superior weight-bearing dome of his acetabulum had been preserved and reduction was accomplished uneventfully, but during the first 3 years after injury he had pain and his result was classified fair. Thereafter his pain subsided so that when last seen, aching and discomfort after dancing were his only symptoms.

Of the 10 patients with fair results, one had a successful reduction on the third attempt 3 days after his injury; one had the hip reduced 48 hours after an amputation above the knee for an ipsilateral open fracture of the leg; and the remaining eight patients had their hips reduced on the day of injury on the first attempt.

In nine of the 23 patients with unsatisfactory results, there were problems in management as follows: A 41-year-old woman's dislocation was not recognized for 5 months and she then had an unsuccessful cup arthroplasty. A 14-year-old child's dislocation (Fig. 3.13), which was associated with an ipsilateral fracture of the femoral shaft, was not recognized until 2 months after injury when roentgenograms to assess the progress of the fractured femur first showed the pelvis. At 10 months an attempt to reduce the dislocated hip by arthrotomy failed because of severe soft tissue contractures. A 23-year-old man had an anterior dislocation on one side and on the other side a posterior fracture-dislocation with an ipsilateral fracture of the femoral shaft. His posterior fracture-dislocation was not recognized and was never reduced (Fig. 3.14). Two patients had redislocations after reduction. One patient had an attempted reduction which was unsuccessful.

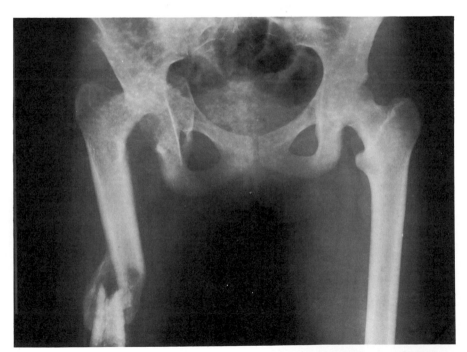

Fig. 3.13 A 14-year-old girl in an automobile accident sustained a type IV fracture-dislocation of the right hip and a fracture of the ipsilateral femur. There was also cerebral concussion with sciatic paralysis. The dislocation of the hip was not recognized until approximately 3 months later, when this roentgenogram of the pelvis was made to determine the progress of the healing femoral fracture. Ten months after injury an attempt was made to reduce the dislocated hip by arthrotomy, but this proved unsuccessful because of severe soft tissue contractures. The result was rated poor. She was last seen at the hospital at the age of 19, when she delivered a normal child.

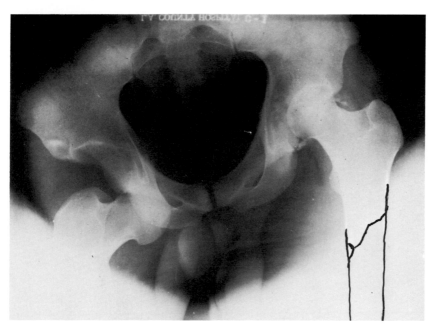

Fig. 3.14 This 23-year-old male sustained an anterior dislocation on the right side and a posterior type IV on the left, together with a fracture of the shaft of the femur and peroneal palsy. The approximate location of the fracture in the diaphysis is indicated by the lines drawn on the roentgenogram. The patient was injured in an auto collision. The posterior dislocation on the side of the femoral shaft fracture was not recognized. Note the fracture of the inner table of the acetabulum at the juncture of the left ischium and relationship with the acetabulum. There are comminuted rim fractures. The results after 5 years and 10 months was found to be excellent for the anterior dislocation. It was poor for the posterior dislocation and there was traumatic arthritis. The peroneal palsy returned to normal by the 12th month.

One patient had a closed reduction accomplished after repeated attempts, but numerous loose bodies were left in the joint; two others had widening of the joint space after closed reduction but the widening was ignored. Of the remaining 14 patients, 11 had their dislocations reduced on the day of injury and three had their dislocations reduced 3 to 4 days after injury.

In all of the 23 hips with poor results, the weight-bearing surface of the acetabulum was damaged. The nature of the injury in type IV fracture-dislocations therefore makes a poor result almost certain because the acetabulum is disrupted.

Type V

In the previous report[26] there was only one good result in a type V hip and at the time of the present study this patient had persistent pain and the rating was reduced to fair. In the 14 type V hips (in 14 patients) included in the present study, there were six fair and eight poor results. Specific factors contributing to these unsatisfactory results were as follows: Two patients had fracture-dislocations that were not recognized. In one of them there was an associated fracture of the neck of the femur, and fusion of the hip was performed at a later late (Fig. 3.15A, B); in the other, the hip lesion was not recognized until 2 1/2 months after injury and a poor result was obtained after a Whitman procedure. A 73-year-old man, on the day of his accident, was scheduled for primary open reduction to remove a loose fragment of the femoral head but during induction he aspirated

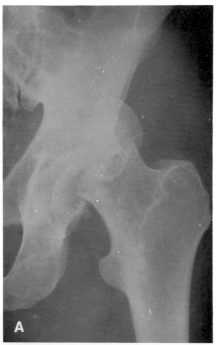

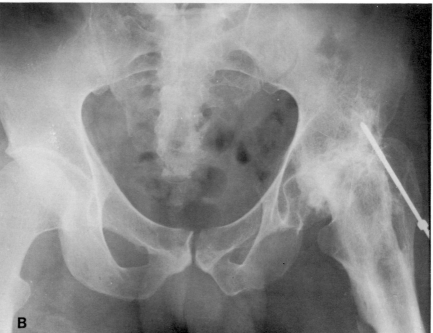

Fig. 3.15   A 29-year-old male sustained this type V posterior dislocation of the left hip when he was involved in an automobile accident. He also had a ruptured spleen and a cerebral concussion. The dislocation was missed and the result was rated poor. *A,* roentgenogram was taken 6 days after injury. First roentgenograms of the hip were not adequate and dislocation was not diagnosed. There is also a subcapital fracture of the hip. *B,* roentgenogram taken 48 months after dislocation reveals a fusion of the hip with a good result.

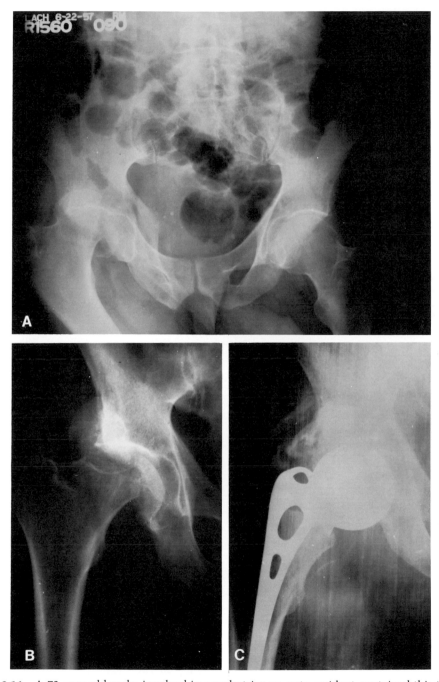

Fig. 3.16 A 73-year-old male, involved in a pedestrian vs. auto accident, sustained this type V dislocation, right, with subsequent fracture of the neck of the femur following closed reduction. Follow-up at 4 months revealed poor result. A, roentgenogram June 22, 1957. Fragment of the femoral head is visible in the acetabulum. There is no evidence of fracture of the neck of the femur. B, roentgenogram June 22, 1957. Patient was taken to surgery on the day of injury for primary open reduction of hip. There was a surgical accident and patient aspirated fluid into lungs. Surgery was canceled. In gentle attempt at closed reduction, the neck of the femur fractured. C, roentgenogram October 29, 1957. Moore prosthesis was inserted 1 week after injury. There is a moderate amount of calcification about the hip joint. Patient walks well with use of cane.

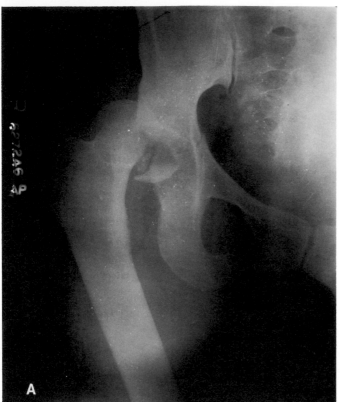

Fig. 3.17 E. S., a 37-year-old woman passenger in an auto vs. auto accident May 12, 1945, her knee striking against the dashboard. She sustained this type V posterior dislocation of her right hip. Twenty-one months later the result was rated poor with traumatic arthritis. *A*, roentgenogram reveals a posterior dislocation with one large and many smaller fragments of the femoral head lying in the acetabulum. *B*, after closed reduction on the day of injury, under general anesthesia. Although on roentgenogram the dislocation appears reduced the avulsed head fragment lies medially alongside the medial portion of the neck. After 2 months of Russell traction, patient started weight-bearing. *C*, roentgenogram shows a diminished joint space. The avulsed head fragment has reattached to the medial portion of the head and neck. Patient has pain and limitation of hip motion.

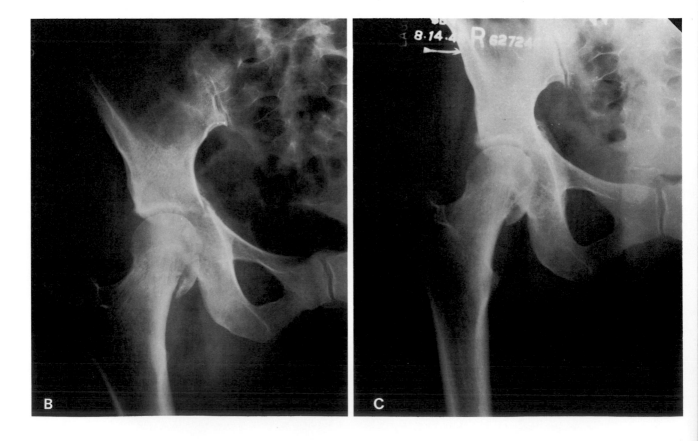

fluid into his lungs and the procedure was canceled. An attempt to reduce the hip by closed manipulation failed and the neck of the femur was fractured during the procedure. One week later an Austin Moore prosthesis was inserted (Fig. 3.16A–C). A 37-year-old woman, whose avulsed femoral head fragment became reattached to the medial portion of the head and neck after reduction, had pain and limitation of hip motion (Fig. 3.17A–C). of the 14 patients 11 had successful manipulative reductions, accomplished within 24 in eight and within 48 hours to 6 weeks after injury in five. In one case multiple attempts at reduction were made; in another, the dislocation reduced spontaneously as the patient was turned on her back after a spinal anesthetic. In general, closed reduction of the dislocation was not a problem in the type V cases, but reduction of the avulsed head fragment was difficult.

CLOSED FOLLOWED BY AN OPEN PROCEDURE

Of the 93 hips treated by closed reduction followed by an open procedure, 13 were type II; 49, type III; 16, type IV; and 15, type V (Table 3.2)

Type II

In the 13 type II hips (in 13 patients) (Figs. 3.18A–C; 3.19A, B; 3.2A–E; 3.21A–C). The results were good in seven, fair in five, and poor in one. Of the seven patients with good results, six had a closed reduction on the day of injury at the first attempt and a delayed open reduction 4 days to 2 months later. In the seventh patient the dislocation was not recognized for 4 days, closed reduction was unsuccessful, and an open procedure was performed on the 5th day. A large fragment of bone, avulsed off the posterior rim of the acetabulum and displaced into the joint, was reduced and fixed with two nails, thereby making the hip stable. In six of these seven hips loose fragments were found in the joint. Of the six patients who had fair or poor results, several had more than one attempt at closed reduction or a greatly delayed open reduction. In one the acetabular fragment was secured with catgut sutures, but within 1 month this fragment was displaced and the hip was subluxated. In the majority of type II cases the avulsed fragments were large, their dimensions ranging from 1×0.75 cm to 8 or 9×3 cm. In most of the unsatisfactory cases the fracture fragment contained articular cartilage.

Table 3.2
Results in 93 Posterior Fracture-Dislocations According to Type: Closed Open Reductions

Type	Good	Fair	Poor	Total	Percentage of good results
II	7	5	1	13	54
III	22	6	21	49	45
IV	5	4	7	16	31
V	5	3	7	15	33
Total	39	18	36	93	41

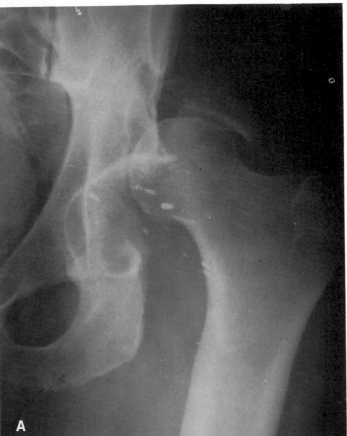

Fig. 3.18 L. A., a 34-year-old man. The roentgenogram shows a type II posterior dislocation. An open reduction was performed 12 days after a closed reduction. The result at 6 months was fair. At 22 years and 10 months the result was good. *A,* roentgenogram made May 29, 1949. Injury was due to an auto collision. The patient also suffered thoracic injuries. A closed reduction was performed on the same day. An open reduction using the posterior approach with replacement of the fractured acetabular fragment was performed on the 12th day. *B,* follow-up roentgenogram taken 6 months later. There was relatively increased density of the central weight-bearing portion of the head with a subchondral depression at its juncture to the atrophic lateral portion of the head. The cartilaginous joint space was still maintained. The patient had pain, muscle spasm, and moderate limitation of hip motion. *C,* roentgenogram made 22 years and 10 months after injury. The result is now rated good. Patient has no pain; however, there is minimal restriction of hip motion. There is no evidence of the subchondral depression of the femoral head. The cartilaginous joint space is still maintained. There is still evidence of areas of increased density throughout the femoral head.

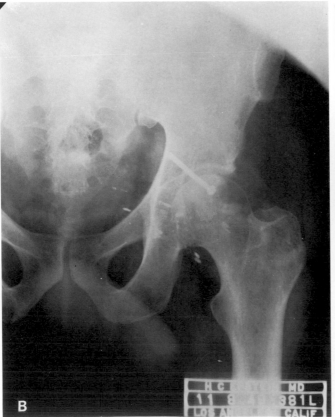

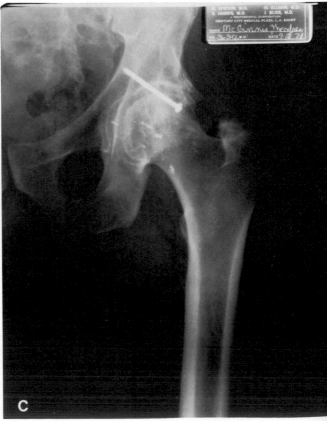

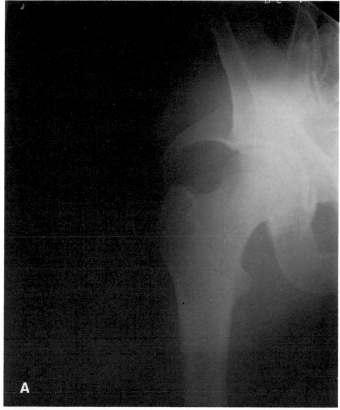

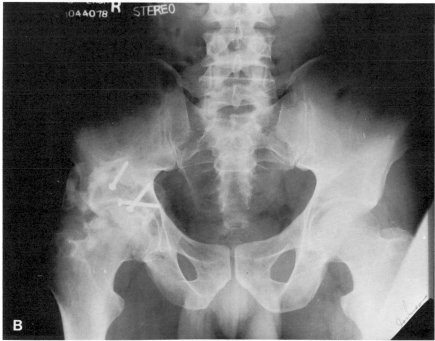

Fig. 3.19 L. J., a 24-year-old male, sustained a posterior type II dislocation of the right hip in a motorcycle accident. The result, 6 months after closed followed by open reduction, was fair with myositis ossificans. *A,* roentgenogram shows reduction with a very large posterior superior acetabular fragment lying posteriorly and superiorly. The reduction under Pentothal anesthesia was difficult. The hip was very unstable and redislocated three times. While in Russell traction the patient's hip was still unstable. *B,* follow-up roentgenogram 6 months after open reduction, performed 8 days after injury. The acetabular fragment measured approximately 8 × 9 × 3cm, and was replaced with difficulty with three screws. There was considerable hemorrhage within the hip joint; the posterior capsule was completely torn. Note the new bone formation about the hip joint with almost complete bridging of the acetabulum to the greater trochanter. Although patient had no pain, there was moderate restriction of hip motion.

131

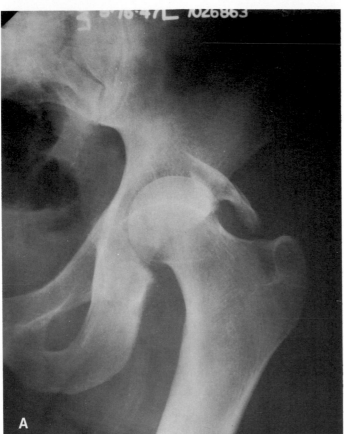

Fig. 3.20   J. C., a 61-year-old male, in an auto vs. streetcar collision, sustained this type II posterior dislocation of his left hip. A closed reduction under spinal anesthesia was performed on the day of injury by the Allis method. An open reduction was performed 2 days later because of hip instability. Progressive changes of avascular necrosis followed over a 1-year period. The result was fair. A, reveals a posterior dislocation of the left hip with a large fragment off the posterior superior acetabular rim. B, after closed reduction the hip appears to be slightly subluxated and the acetabular fragment is displaced. C, check roentgenogram 3 months after an open reduction was accomplished (2 days after injury). A posterior approach was used. Blood clots and debris were removed from the hip joint. The large fragment (1½ cm long by 1 cm wide and 4 mm thick) of avulsed bone was curetted and reattached to the acetabulum with suture of No.1 chromic. A one and one-half spica cast was applied for 2 months. Full weight-bearing was not permitted for 6 months. Note that the fragment has displaced.

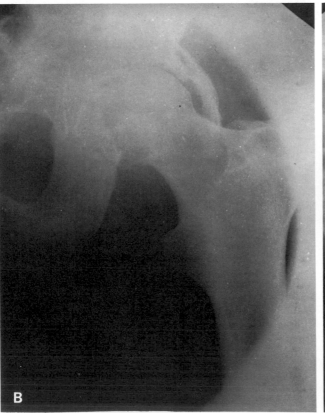

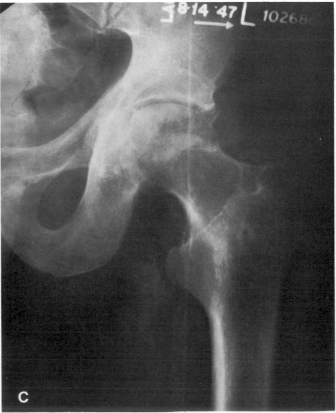

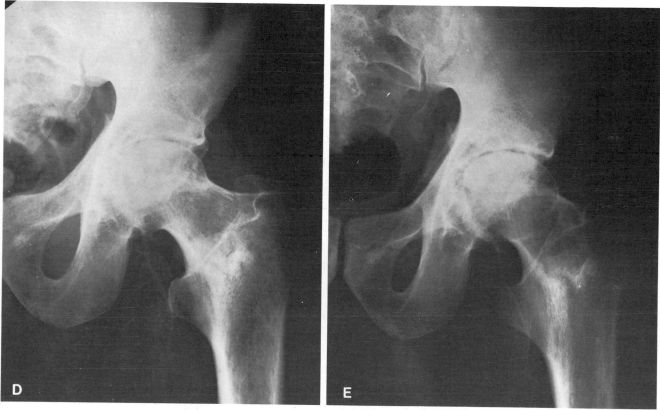

Fig. 3.20 *D,* five months after reduction, there is the first indication of narrowing of the hip joint which usually occurs with traumatic arthritis. Patient has moderate limitation of hip motion with minimal pain. He uses crutches for weight-bearing. *E,* roentgenograms taken at 6 months and 1 year reveal the progressive changes of avascular necrosis. There are areas of increased and decreased densities throughout the femoral head.

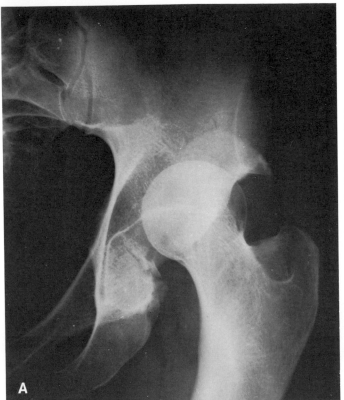

Fig. 3.21 In this 35-year-old patient, the roentgenogram shows a posterior dislocation, type II, on which an open reduction was performed. Avascular necrosis developed and the result was poor. A, the patient was injured in a collision of an auto and truck. A closed reduction was performed the same day. B, roentgenogram made after the closed reduction. An open reduction was performed 7 days later. C, follow-up roentgenogram after 3 years and 7 months. Patient had disabling pain, muscle spasm and severe limitation of hip motion. Note the central depression in the dense fragment of the femoral head and the mottled cancellous bone of the head with bone production at the margins of the head and neck; superiorly there is still a fair but irregular cartilaginous space but medially it is thin.

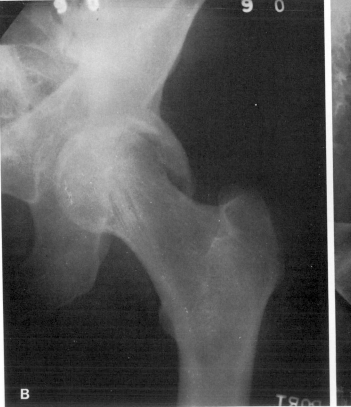

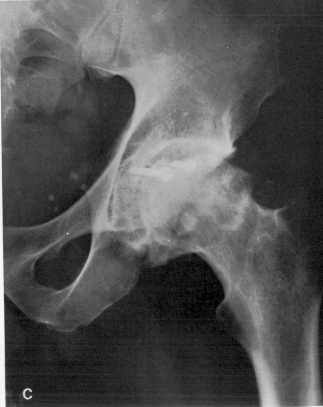

Type III

In the 49 type III hips (in 49 patients) there were 22 good, six fair, and 21 poor results (Figs. 3.22*A*, *B*; 3.23*A*, *B*; 3.24*A*, *B*). In the 22 good results the hips were redislocated and the joint spaces were meticulously checked for loose fragments of bone and cartilage. In one patient whose hip was unstable after closed reduction and in another in whom manipulation failed, open reduction was performed on the day of injury. Three patients had closed followed by open reduction 5, 7, and 8 days later, all with good results. In the remaining patients (all with loose fragments in the hip joint) closed and open reductions were performed within 24 hours after injury. In two, fixation of the avulsed fragments was impossible because the fragments were too small, but the results were good nonetheless.

Twenty-seven of the fair or poor results were associated with a postoperative infection in four, an unsuccessful closed followed by an open procedure in four, redislocations of the hip after closed reduction followed by an open procedure in two, and failure to remove all fragments from the hip joint in two (Fig. 3.25*A*–*C*).

Significant findings in the other unsatisfacatory results included: a long delay between the open and closed reduction (ranging from 3 weeks to 2 months) in six; penetration of the femoral head by a screw used to fix the acetabular fragment in one; delayed open reduction because of a decubitus ulcer on the buttock on the involved side in one; an anterior approach for removal of loose fragments approximately 1 month after a closed reduction in two; and no reduction of the dislocation in five.

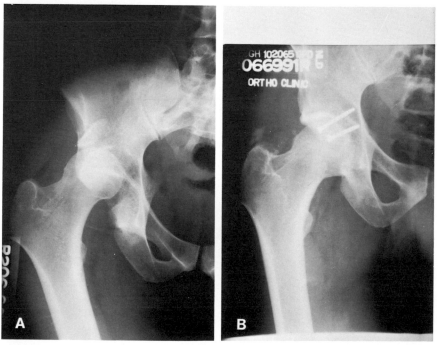

Fig. 3.22 A 33-year-old male in auto vs. train accident, in poor condition with pneumothorax. Hip was unstable after closed reduction in flexion. Open reduction was done the same day with removal of small fragments from hip joint. A large acetabular fragment was repositioned with two screws. Patient was in traction for 6 weeks; weight-bearing at 4 months. Result, 4½ years later, is good.

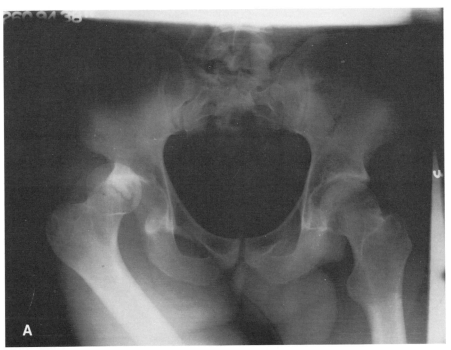

Fig. 3.23 A 23-year-old male was in an auto vs. bus accident and sustained a type III posterior dislocation of his right hip. The patient was in shock and had an injury to his chest. A closed reduction was done on the day of injury, and 2 days later an open reduction was performed. The result 12 months after injury was poor with avascular necrosis. A, roentgenogram reveals posterior dislocation with multiple fragments.

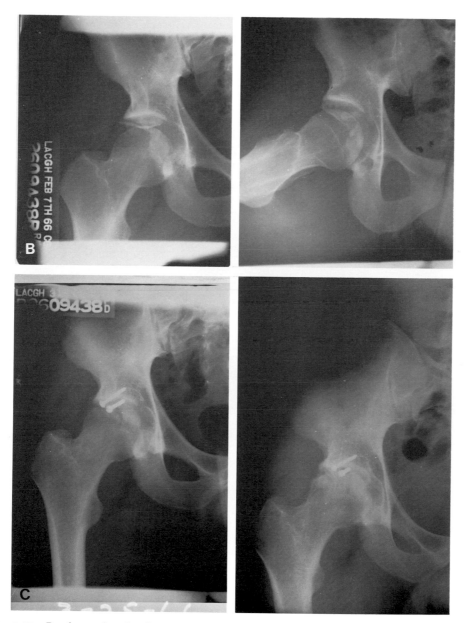

Fig. 3.23 *B,* after a closed reduction on the day of injury there are fragments within the hip joint, which is unstable. *C,* roentgenogram taken 7 months after open reduction. Many fragments were removed from the joint space and the larger posterior rim fragment was transfixed with two screws. The lower screw appears to be through the femoral head. Patient has had persistent hip pain since his discharge. One month after injury avascular necrosis is evident.

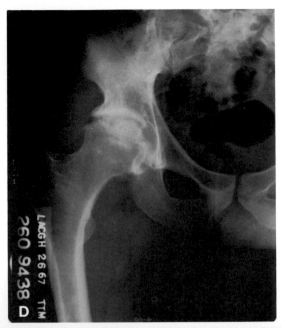

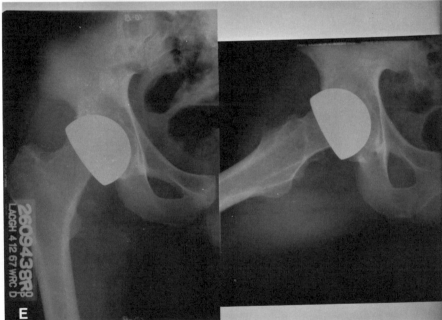

Fig. 3.23 *D,* one year after open reduction both screws were removed. The lower screw had penetrated the femoral head cartilage. *E,* a cup arthroplasty was performed 14 months after injury. The result at 19 months was good.

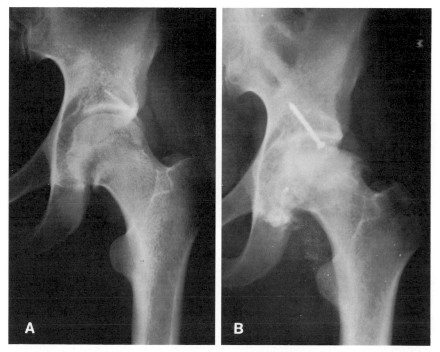

Fig. 3.24 This 27-year-old man involved in an auto accident dislocated his left hip, sustaining this type III posterior dislocation. A closed reduction was done in another city; an open reduction was performed at the USC/LAC Medical Center 3 days later. The result at 28 months was rated poor with avascular necrosis. *A*, roentgenogram on day of admission. The dislocation has been reduced. Many fragments appear to be within the hip joint. *B*, roentgenogram 38 months after injury. At surgery there was considerable trauma to the hip. There were many loose fragments removed from the hip joint. The capsule was shredded; there were thrombosed veins and arteries as well as torn short rotator muscles. The posterior acetabular rim was transfixed with one screw. Note the avascular necrosis with flattening and irregularity of the femoral head. There was marked limitation of the hip with considerable pain. The patient stated he wanted his hip fused.

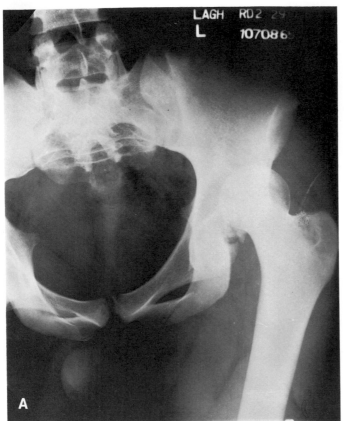

Fig. 3.25 This 18-year-old male was in a truck vs. auto accident, sustaining this type III posterior fracture-dislocation. The result 10 months later was fair with traumatic arthritis. *A,* note the absence of the lessor trochanter and the multiple fragments about the hip joint. *B,* a closed performance was done on the day of injury using the Allis method. Note the wide joint space with a bony fragment within the hip joint. *C,* at surgery 2 days after injury, three fragments were removed, two lying outside of the joint and one within the joint space. The fragments were too small for fixation to the acetabulum. *The hip was not redislocated to check for smaller fragments.* Note the small fragment within the hip joint causing an incongruity, a definite cause of traumatic arthritis.

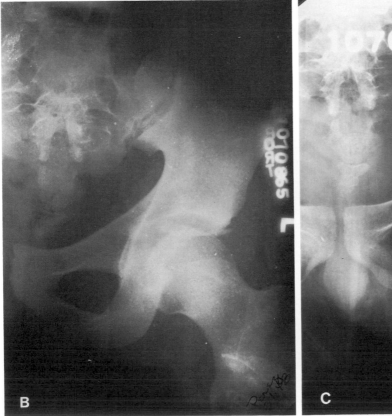

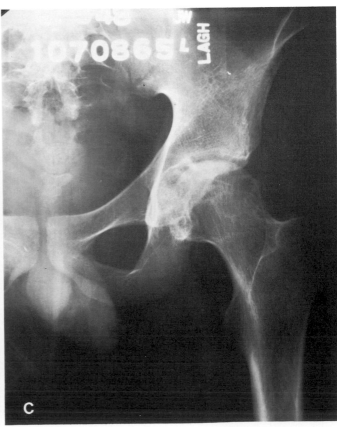

Type IV

In the 16 type IV hips (in 16 patients) there were five good, four fair, and seven poor results (Figs. 3.26A–D; 3.27A–C). Of the five good results, two were in patients whose open procedure was done 10 and 25 days after injury, and two were in patients who had bilateral hip injury with a type IV lesion on one side and an anterior dislocation on the other. The fifth good result followed an open procedure done 2 days after a closed reduction. In all of these five hips no attempt was made to fix the fragments in the floor of the acetabulum, but the main posterior rim fragments were fixed either with screws or with nails. Loose fragments were found in three of these five hips.

In four patients with fair results one had an unsuccessful closed followed by an open reduction 2 days later, and in the other three patients the hips were opened 2, 8, and 14 days after a closed reduction—the latter because the patient was comatose (Fig. 3.28A–C).

In three of the seven patients with poor results, arthrotomy using an anterior approach was performed 10 days, 4 weeks, and 6 weeks after injury to remove loose fragments from the joint in two, and to correct hip flexion contractures in the third. In the other three patients the dislocation could not be reduced by closed methods. In the first of these, the obturator internus muscle was wrapped around the neck of the femur and the dislocation could be reduced only after the tendon was severed at its attachment to the trochanter. In addition, there was a large fragment of acetabulum including articular cartilage (2 × 2 cm) with no soft tissue attachments, as well as numerous smaller fragments in the joint. Fragments of cartilage and bone from the medial and posterior portion of the femoral head were also removed. In the second patient, in whom closed reduction was not possible, three large fragments in the hip joint prevented reduction and at operation replacement and fixation of the fragments was not possible. In the third patient, with irreducible fracture dislocation, there was an ipsilateral fracture of the femoral shaft as well as complete disruption of the posterior rim and floor of the acetabulum; a total hip replacement was performed 9 months later. In the last case, the hip became infected following open reduction.

Type V

In the 15 type V hips (in 15 patients) there were five good, three fair, and seven poor results. In the five patients with good results, closed reduction was successful in one and unsuccessful in four, despite three attempts in one of them. The open procedures in these five patients were performed on the day of the injury in two, 28 hours after injury in one and on the 1st day of hospitalization in the other (this patient had apparently been lying unconscious in an overturned car for 1 to 3 days). The lesser fragment of the femoral head, which in each instance included approximately one-fourth to one-third of the head, was excised. This fragment, which was lying in the acetabulum, probably prevented closed reduction of three of the four hips. The ligamentum teres was attached to the main fragment in two instances. Numerous smaller fragments were removed from the acetabulum in all five patients.

In the 10 unsatisfactory cases there were several features that appeared to have contributed to the unsatisfactory results. The secondary procedure was done through an anterior approach in six patients (one fair and five poor results. In addition, one of these six patients had a concurrent fracture of the ipsilateral femoral neck and another required hip fusion for pain 9 months after exploration.

Of the other three patients with unsatisfactory results, two had the lesser head fragment approximated to the main fragment of the femoral head with no attempt at rigid internal fixation; one had approximately the medial half of the weight-

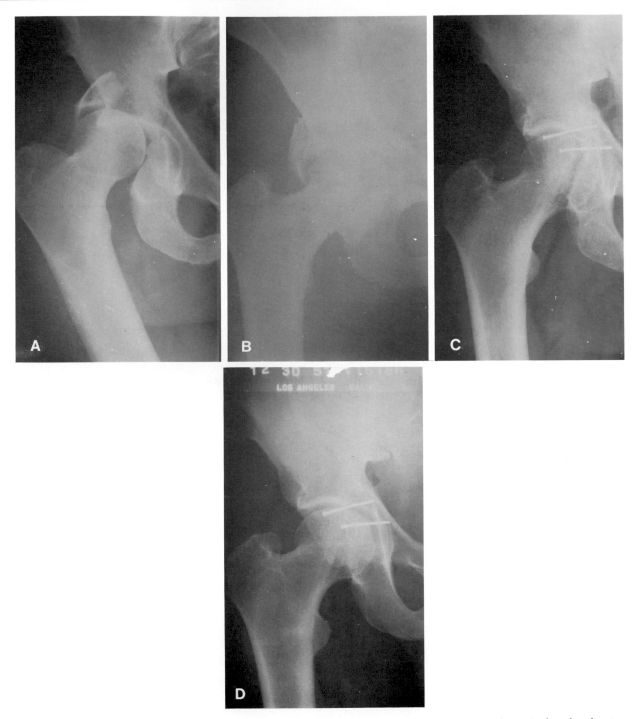

Fig. 3.26   A 49-year-old male sustained this type IV posterior dislocation in an automobile accident. A closed reduction was done 1 day after his injury followed by an open reduction 25 days later. The result was rated good at 7-year follow-up, *A*, roentgenogram on day of admission. There is a fracture of the posterior superior acetabular rim with a fracture through the flow of the acetabulum with minimum displacement. *B*, roentgenogram after reduction. The superior rim fracture is displaced laterally. The femoral head does not appear to have penetrated medially. *C*, roentgenogram after reduction. The superior rim fracture is displaced laterally. The femoral head does not appear to have penetrated medially. *C*, roentgenogram 8 months after open reduction, performed 25 days after injury. The acetabular fragment was transfixed with two stainless steel nails. No attempt was made to transfix the fracture through the roof of the acetabulum. No mention was made of loose fragments within the joint. *D*, roentgenogram 7 years after injury. There is no avascular necrosis or traumatic arthritis. The joint space is normal. Patient has 10° limitation of internal and external rotation of the right hip; otherwise motion is normal. Patient has never had any hip pain and has been doing heavy work without any discomfort. Hip occasionally feels tired after a day's work.

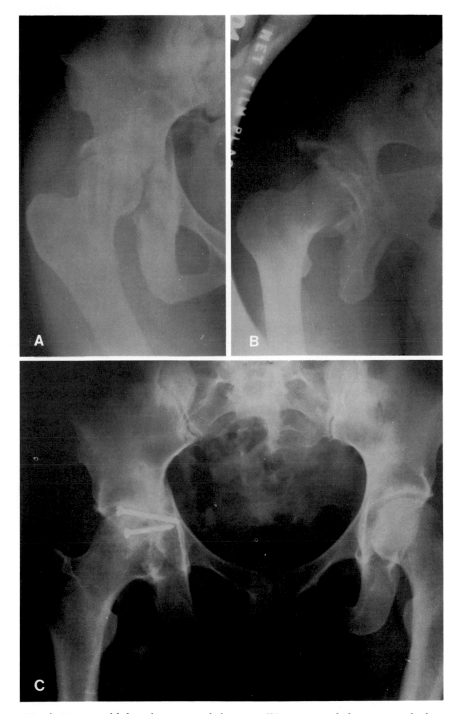

Fig. 3.27 A 39-year-old female sustained this type IV posterior dislocation, right hip, in a collision between auto and fire plug. Good result. *A,* roentgenogram on day of injury. Note that the fracture involves weight-bearing portion of floor and rim of acetabulum. *B,* after closed reduction, same day. This resembles a central protrusion fracture of acetabulum. *C,* open reduction 2 days later. There were loose fragments in the joint. Roentgenograms 54 months after injury show that the joint space is normal. Patient has normal gait without limp. There is 15° flexion contracture and 15° limitation of internal rotation of the hip.

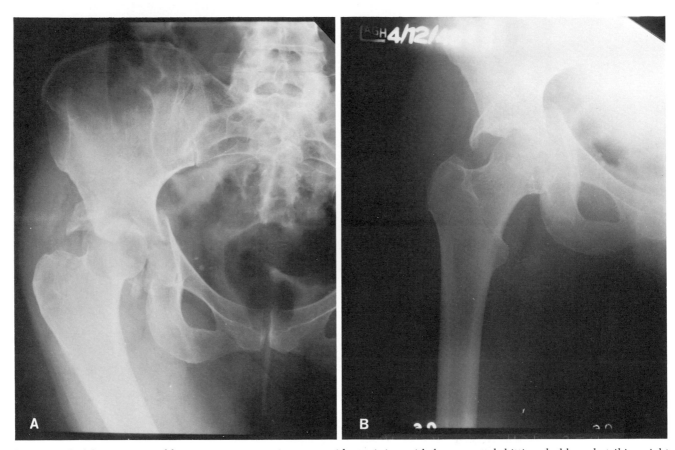

Fig. 3.28 L. M., a 51-year-old woman passenger in auto accident, sitting with legs crossed, hitting dashboard striking right patella, sustained a type IV dislocation. *A,* she did not wear a seatbelt. There was a temporary period of unconsciousness. Note the large fragment off the posterior acetabular rim and fractures through the floor of the acetabulum. *B,* a closed reduction was performed on the day of injury easily under general anesthetic (see color photographs of reduction, Fig. 7.2), and Russell traction was applied.

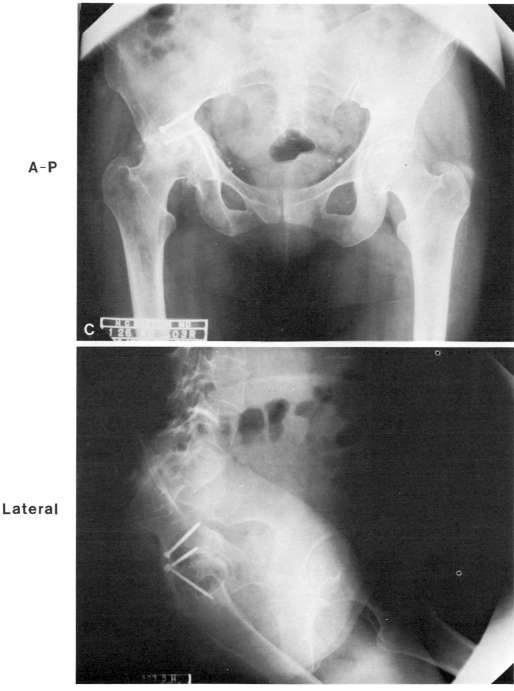

Fig. 3.28 *C,* the hip was unstable after reduction. However, an open reduction was delayed for 12 days because of a severe ileus. A posterior approach was made. There was considerable old hemorrhage along the inferior portion of the gluteus maximus muscle and the tensor fascia lata. The sciatic nerve was found lying over the fragments of the acetabulum floor but was not injured. All the short rotators except the piriformis were in one large mass and appeared to have been injured and had organized granulation tissue and hematoma. There was a large stellate tear in the posterior capsule. An attempt was made to approximate the ilium and ischium with one screw and this held fairly well. The avulsed fracture of the posterior rim of the acetabulum was replaced anatomically with two screws. There were many loose portions of bone which were removed from the hip joint itself. This left a short gap in the acetabulum approximately ½ inch wide between the ischium and posterior lip. The head of the femur showed numerous compressions involving the articular surfaces. Fourteen months after injury, anterior-posterior and lateral views reveal the three screws used for fixation. There is early avascular necrosis with areas of increased and decreased densities. Although patient does not have hip pain she needs crutches for support. Motions of the hip is limited to approximately 50% of normal. At this time the result was rated fair.

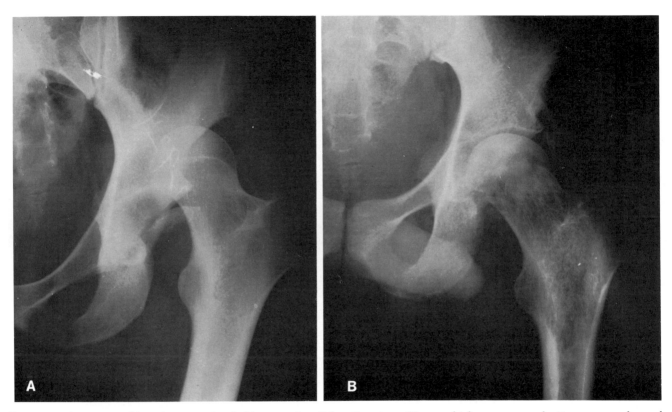

Fig. 3.29 A 22-year-old patient sustained this posterior dislocation, type V, on which an open reduction was performed. Avascular necrosis developed and the result was poor. *A,* The patient was injured in an auto collision. There was also a fracture in the proximal third of the ipsilateral tibia with circulatory impairment. Note the free fragment of the head of the femur. The dislocation was irreducible by closed manipulation; an open reduction was performed 3 weeks after injury. *B,* roentgenogram made about 3 months after open reduction. The acetabular labrum was folded over the acetabulum and prevented closed reduction. The fragment from the fractured head was not removed. There was sufficient atrophy of the proximal portion of the femur to show the unchanged density of the head.

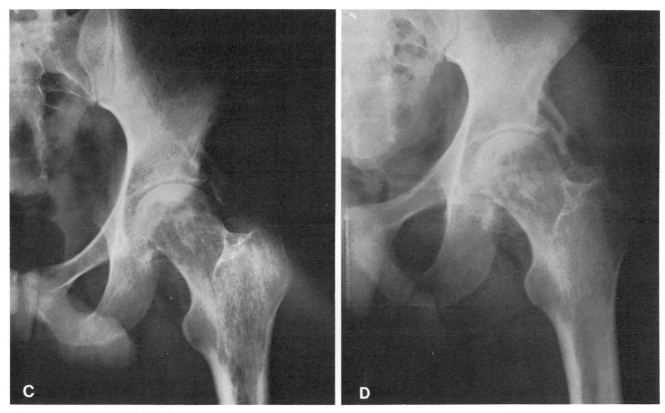

Fig. 3.29 *C*, roentgenogram made 5 months after reduction. Note the general atrophy, especially of the upper end of the femur, except for the lunate area of increased density at the weight-bearing portion of the head. Capsular calcification is evident. *D*, roentgenogram made 1 year later. Note the increased calcification and the spreading of irregular areas of increased density at the weight-bearing portion of the head. The cartilaginous joint space is narrowed. The patient had pain and limitation of hip motion.

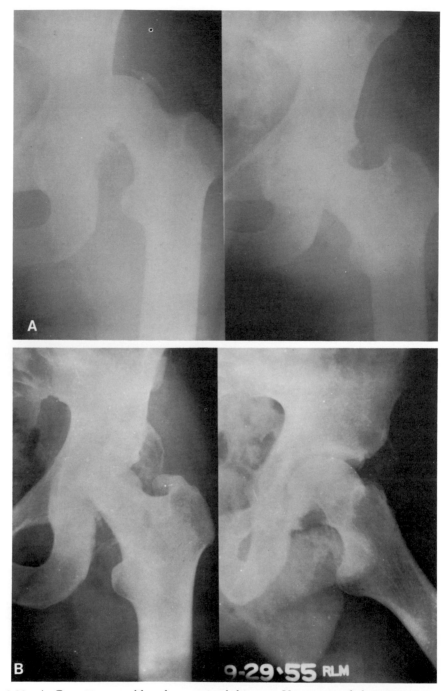

Fig. 3.30 A. G., a 32-year-old male, sustained this type V posterior dislocation. in an auto accident, August 20, 1955. *A,* roentgenogram on day of injury. There is a portion of bone lying inferiorly and superiorly which appears to be off of the femoral head. *B,* reduction by closed method is apparent, after two unsuccessful attempts. Open reduction was performed 4 days later, with removal of one-half of the medial weight-bearing portion of the head. The fragment was 2 inches in diameter and 1 inch thick.

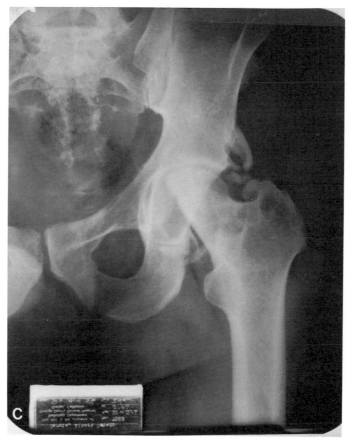

Fig. 3.30 C, roentgenogram 1 year later. There is a minimal amount of soft tissue calcification about the hip joint. The medial inferior portion of the head, involving a good amount of the weight-bearing portion, has been removed. There is no evidence of avascular necrosis in the remaining portion of the head, and the joint space is normal. The stresses on his hip are now too great for the patient to bear asymptomatically. He has pain and was unable to continue with his work as a hod carrier.

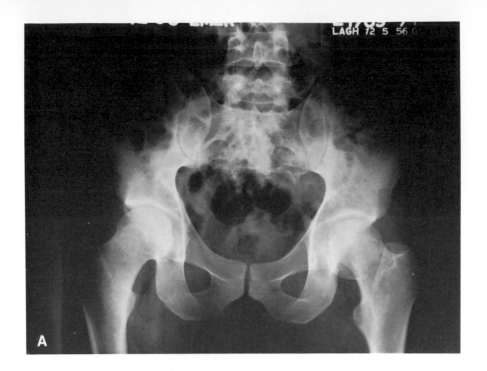

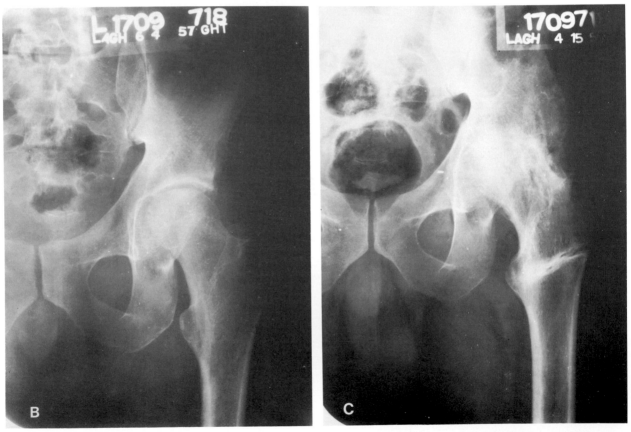

Fig. 3.31 N. C., a 31-year-old male, driver of an automobile that went over an embankment on December 1, 1956, sustained this type V dislocation of the left hip. The result, 10 months after a closed followed by an open reduction, using an anterior approach, was rated poor with fusion of the hip. *A*, roentgenogram reveals reduction of the dislocation, showing the fracture of the inferior portion of the head. *B*, this roentgenogram shows the hip 10 days after an anterior approach was made to remove the fragment, which consisted of one-third of the articular surface of the head with its attachment to the ligamentum teres. Pain has been persistent in the hip since the patient started weight-bearing at 2 months. *C*, because of persistent pain and disability, the hip was fused 10 months after patient's injury. An iliac bone graft was used for the fusion with a transverse subtrochanteric osteotomy performed. The hip was solidly fused on May 9, 1958.

Table 3.3
Results in 83 Posterior Fracture-Dislocations According to Type: Primary Open
Reduction

Type	Good	Fair	Poor	Total	Percentage of good results
II	7	1	0	8	87
III	29	7	7	43	67
IV	6	4	5	15	40
V	8	2	7	17	47
Total	50	14	19	83	60

bearing surface of the head removed, with a poor result because the hip was too
unstable for the patient to continue his occupation as a hod carrier (Figs. 3.29A–
D; 3.30A–C; 3.31A–C). In the other poor result there was an infection.

PRIMARY OPEN REDUCTION

Of the 83 hips treated by primary open reduction, eight were type II; 43, type
III; 15, type IV; 17, type V (Table 3.3).

Type II

In the eight type II hips (in eight patients) there were seven good results and
one fair result (Figs. 3.32A, B; 3.33A–C). Of these eight hips, one was operated on
2 days after injury with a good result; the other seven were operated on within 24
hours after injury. Small bone fragments, most of them not visible on rooentgen-
ograms, were found in seven of the eight hips. In the other hip, the joint space
was irrigated with saline but no mention was made of loose fragments.

At follow-up the patient with the fair result had some pain and traumatic
arthritis, as indicated by narrowing of the joint space. One of the two screws used
to fix the acetabular fragment had backed out with resultant lateral displacement
of the fragment.

Type III

In the 43 type III hips (in 43 patients) the results were good in 29, fair in seven,
and poor in seven. Among the good results the operations were performed within
24 hours after injury in all but two hips. In these two, open procedures were done
5 and 13 days after injury, but the results were good (Figs. 3.34A, B; 3.35A, B).
Fragments of bone or cartilage were removed from 37 of the 43 hips. No fragments
were found in two, and the operative notes failed to comment on fragments in the
other four. Acetabular fragments too small to be fixed internally were left *in situ*
in six hips, four with good and two with fair results.

Of the seven fair results, two were in the hips mentioned previously with small
acetabular fragments left *in situ* without internal fixation. Follow-up roentgenograms of these seven type III hips showed narrowing of the cartilage space
consistent with traumatic arthritis.

The seven poor results were as follows: One patient died of cardiac arrest
during operation. Three patients had postoperative infections. One of the infections was in a 77-year-old man whose hip dislocated, was reduced with traction,
and then redislocated, whereupon no further attempt was made to relocate it.
The second infected hip occurred in a 47-year-old diabetic man with an ipsilateral
fracture of the femoral shaft. The femur was first internally fixed with an

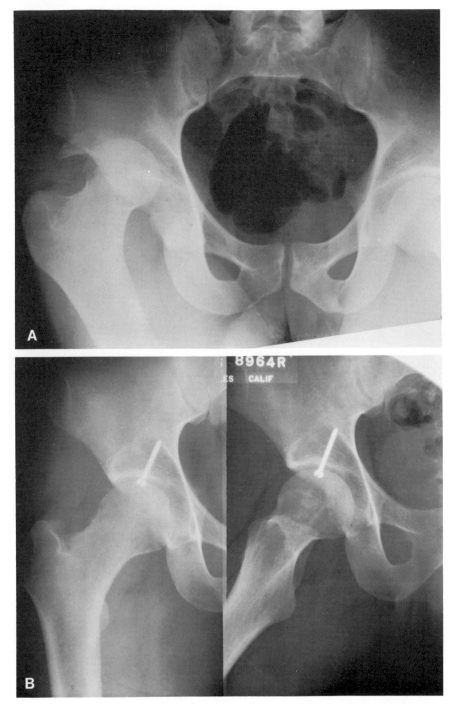

Fig. 3.32 O. R., a 24-year-old male, was injured in an auto accident on April 18, 1954. This type II dislocation, right, was treated by open reduction. Follow-up at 46 months showed good result. Patient also sustained a middle fossa skull fracture with cerebral concussion. *A*, there is a large fragment off the posterior superior acetabular rim. No smaller fragments are visualized. *B*, roentgenograms taken June 28, 1956; primary open reduction on day of injury. Although not visualized by roentgenograms, small fragments were removed from the hip joint. The hip joint appears normal with one screw transfixing the acetabular rim fracture. There was minimal limitation only in internal rotation of the hip. The patient has no hip or knee pain and works regularly as a draftsman.

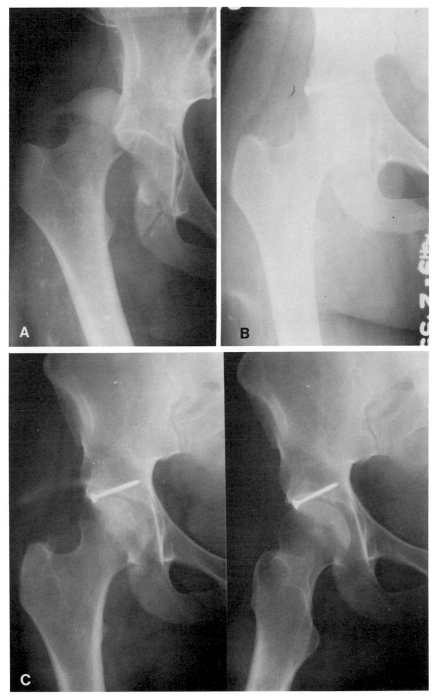

Fig. 3.33 L. S., a 33-year-old female involved in an auto accident. This type II posterior dislocation, right, was treated by primary open reduction on day of accident. Follow-up at 35 months showed good result. *A*, roentgenograms February 3, 1955. Note the large posterior superior acetabular rim. There are no small fragments visualized in the joint. *B*, roentgenograms September 2, 1955 (7 months after surgery). Two small fragments were removed from the hip joint. One screw transfixed the large acetabular fragment. Stability of the hip joint was good. *C*, roentgenograms January 4, 1958 (anterior and posterior). There is normal joint space, no avascular necrosis or traumatic arthritis. No calcification is seen. There is a small loose fragment which lies in the inferior medial border of the hip joint. Internal and external rotation are limited 10°. The rest of the motions are normal. Patient has never had any pain and no limp. She was kept in traction 6 weeks and walked with crutches at 2½ months without weight-bearing.

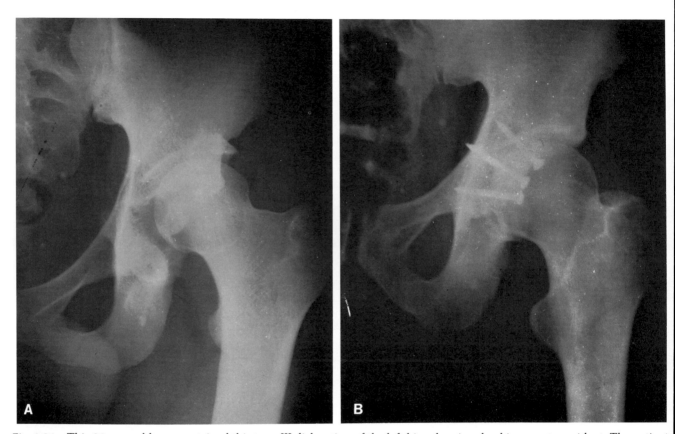

Fig. 3.34   This 21-year-old man sustained this type III dislocation of the left hip when involved in an auto accident. The patient was unconscious for 5 days and no attempt was made at closed reduction. On the 5th day an open reduction was performed with removal of three fragments of bone from the hip joint. At follow-up, 5 years and 10 months after injury, the result was rated good. *A*, roentgenogram made on day of injury. *B*, roentgenogram made at follow-up. The patient had no pain but there was slight limitation of hip motion. There is no evidence of traumatic arthritis or avascular necrosis.

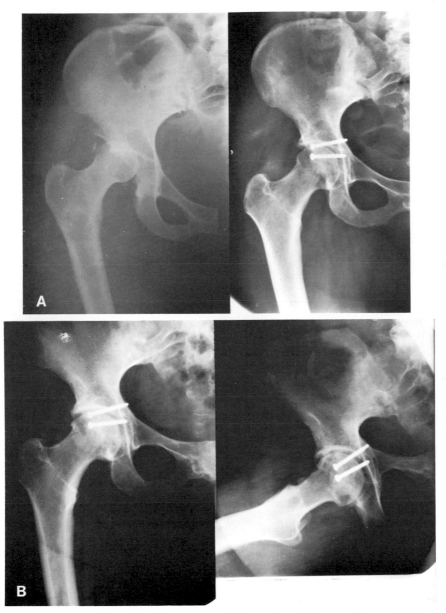

Fig. 3.35 A 38-year-old woman after an automobile accident had a type III posterior fracture-dislocation of the right hip. Primary open reduction was performed 13 days after injury. Many small fragments were removed and a large fragment from the posterior rim was replaced and fixed with two screws. The limb was maintained in traction for 2 months and the patient started weight-bearing in 3 months. Nineteen years after injury the patient had no pain and a good range of hip motion. *A,* before and after reduction. *B,* at follow-up the joint space is normal with no evidence of avascular necrosis. On the superior margin of the head and neck there is minimal spur formation.

intramedullary rod and then the fracture-dislocation of the hip was reduced after many small fragments were removed from the joint. The larger fragments of the acetabular rim were left *in situ*. This patient had a sciatic neve paralysis (which had not returned to normal after 15 months), but no contusion of the sciatic nerve was found at surgery. The infection started first in the femur and spread to the hip joint after the intramedullary rod was removed. Drainage persisted for 15 months after injury. The third infection was still draining 14 months after surgery.

The remaining three patients with poor results included two whose hips subluxated at 8 and 10 months, respectively, and the last case occurred in a 50-year-old woman who had severe traumatic arthritis 9½ years after injury. Many bone fragments which appeared to come from the acetabular rim were found in her hip; however, no fixation was possible because the fragments were too small. Although peroneal nerve paralysis was present and did not return to normal, the condition of the nerve at surgery was not mentioned.

Type IV

In the 15 type IV hips (in 15 patients) the results were good in six, fair in four, and poor in two (Figs. 3.36*A*, *B*; 3.37*A–C*). All of these hips were operated on less than 24 hours after injury and fragments were found in all but five of the joints (Fig. 3.38*A–C*). Although no mention was made of the presence or absence of loose fragments in these five hips, they were thoroughly irrigated with saline.

It is difficult to explain the different results in the six good, four fair, and five poor cases. Of the six patients with good results, five had internal fixation and one simple removal of a loose fragment and reduction of the dislocation. Of the four with fair results, one had extensive contusions of the femoral head and subsequent traumatic arthritis, and three had small chip fractures of the femoral head (not fixed in two and held with catgut sutures in one).

One of the five patients with poor results was a 52-year-old man who had fragments too small for internal fixation. At follow-up 30 months after injury roentgenograms revealed avascular necrosis of the femoral head. Another patient, a 67-year-old woman, had subluxation 10 days after reduction when the traction was removed because she was constantly moving about and removing the traction herself. Both moderate traumatic arthritis and moderate myositis ossificans were evident 1 year after injury.

In two, the hips were rated as fair but this was changed to poor because of severe traumatic arthritis in one and myositis ossificans in the other. Both patients had painful hips on weight-bearing at the time of follow-up. In the last patient with a poor result a deep infection followed surgery.

The surgical procedure in all but one of the type IV hips was limited to removal of loose pieces of bone, reduction of the dislocation, and fixation of the posterior rim (when possible) to gain stability and restore as normal an acetabular-femoral head relationship as possible. In the one exception, a hip with extensive comminution of the acetabulum and posterior dislocation, fragments were reduced and then after reduction of the dislocation these fragments were internally fixed with a plate and screws with a good result.

Type V

In the 17 type V (in 17 patients) there were eight good, two fair, and seven poor results (Figs. 3.39*A*, *B*; 3.40*A-C*; 3.41*A*, *B*). Three of the 17 patients were operated on 6, 8, and 17 days after injury. The other 14 had their operations within 24 hours after injury. In four of these hips the femoral neck was fractured as well as the femoral head. Treatment in these four cases was as follows: In one, the lesser

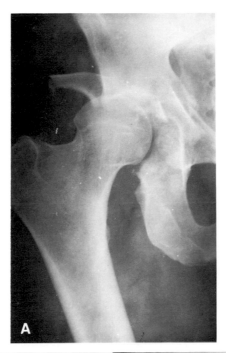

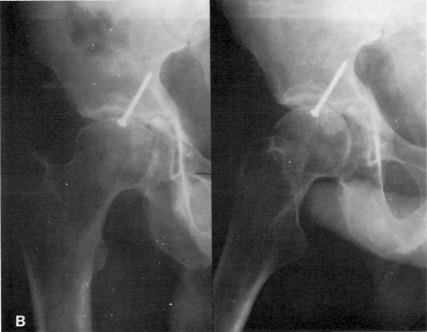

Fig. 3.36 A man, 39 years old, sustained a type IV posterior dislocation of the right hip with peroneal palsy in an automobile accident. Primary open reduction was performed and the result was rated good. *A*, roentgenogram made on day of injury shows a large fracture of the posterior superior acetabular rim extending through the floor and rim of the acetabulum. *B*, anterior-posterior and lateral roentgenograms made 54 months later. At primary open reduction there were many loose fragments in the joint. The large acetabular rim fracture was transfixed with one screw but no attempt was made to transfix the fracture through the floor of the acetabulum. At last follow-up the peroneal nerve paralysis had recovered completely, there was minimum restriction of motion of the hip, and the patient was working regularly as a salesman, free of hip pain.

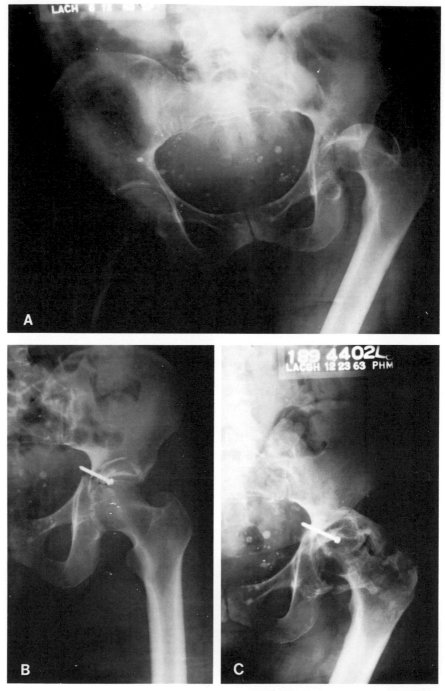

Fig. 3.37 F. C., a 67-year-old woman, was struck by an automobile, sustaining this type IV fracture-dislocation of the left hip with peroneal palsy. Patient had a primary open reduction. One year later the result was rated poor. *A*, there is a posterior dislocation with a fracture through the floor and roof of the acetabulum. *B*, roentgenogram made after a primary open reduction was performed on the day of injury. There was no mention made of the condition of the peroneal nerve. Many fragments were removed from the hip joint. One screw transfixed the acetabular fragment. No attempt was made to stabilize the floor of the acetabulum. *C*, this roentgenogram reveals the hip 6 months after surgery. There is moderate myositis ossificans with subluxation of the hip joint. Patient became confused because of cerebral ischemia and repeatedly removed her traction. The traction was finally removed 9 days after surgery with the hip subluxating. When last seen 1 year after injury, patient had a complete peroneal paralysis and she was unable to walk without assistance.

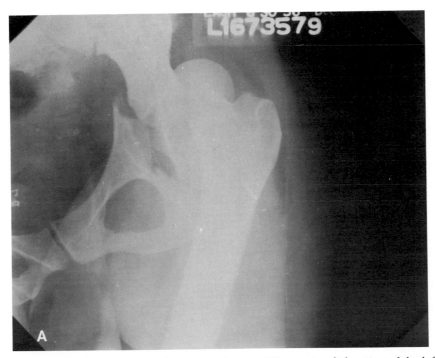

Fig. 3.38 E. M., a 39-year-old female, sustained a type IV posterior dislocation of the left hip in an automobile collision. Primary open reduction was performed the day of injury. At follow-up the result was rated poor, with avascular necrosis of the femoral head. *A*, roentgenogram made on June 30, 1956, the day of injury, reveals a fracture through the floor and rim of the acetabulum.

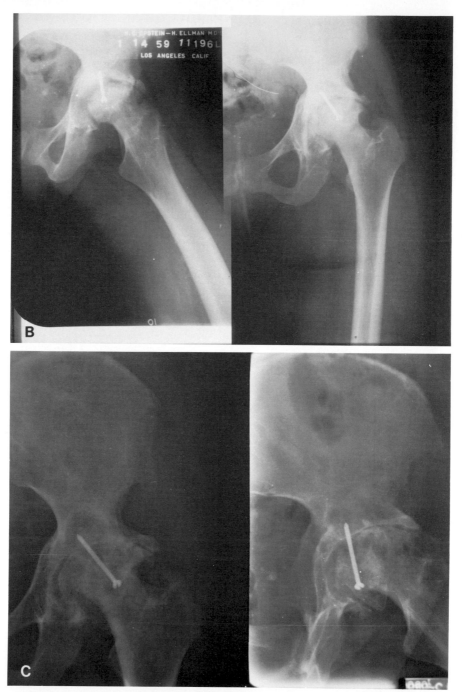

Fig. 3.38 *B,* roentgenograms made on January 14, 1959, 30 months after injury, show moderate narrowing of the joint space with a depression over the weight-bearing portion of the femoral head and areas of increased and decreased densities. At open reduction, the day of injury, one screw was used to transfix the large acetabular fracture of the posterior rim; no attempt was made to reduce the fracture through the floor of the acetabulum. At the time these roentgenograms were made the patient walked with a limp and had limited motion of the hip. There was numbness in the left great toe which had persisted since the accident but there was no weakness in the muscles of the foot. Three months later, at the last follow-up, she was walking much better, using a cane. *C,* roentgenograms made in August 1973, more than 17 years after her original injury. Moderately severe degenerative changes are noted throughout the left hip joint involving both the femoral head and the acetabular component. This is a sequela of the avascular necrosis that occurred after her surgery. The patient was having a moderate amount of hip pain and used a cane for weight-bearing. There was a moderate amount of limitation of motion. Patient was being considered for a total hip prosthesis in the near future.

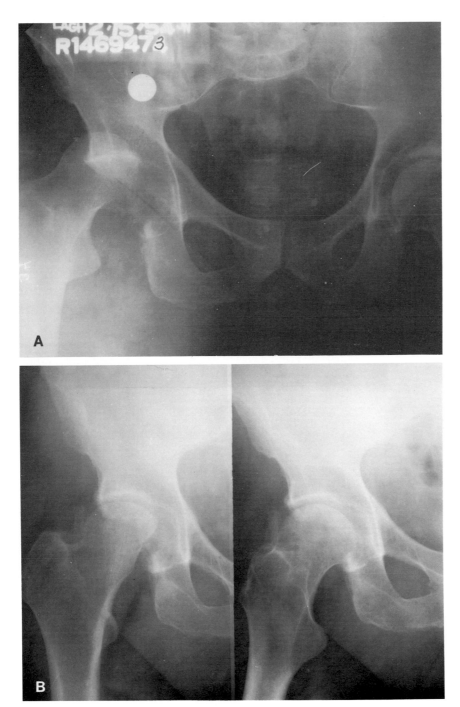

Fig. 3.39 R. C., a 44-year-old male, with type V dislocation, right, treated by primary open reduction. Follow-up at 8½ years showed good results. *A*, roentgenogram, February 15, 1954. Approximately one-fourth of the inferior medial portion of the femoral head was removed. This was lying in the acetabulum and was attached to the ligamentum teres. There were also smaller fragments removed from the joint. Patient was in traction for 1 month and used crutches with weight-bearing for 2 weeks. *B*, roentgenograms (anterior-posterior and lateral), December 15, 1957. There is minimal calcification superiorly. Approximately one-fourth of the head is missing inferiorly. Joint space is normal. There is no avascular necrosis. Patient does not have pain and works regularly. There is good motion of the hip.

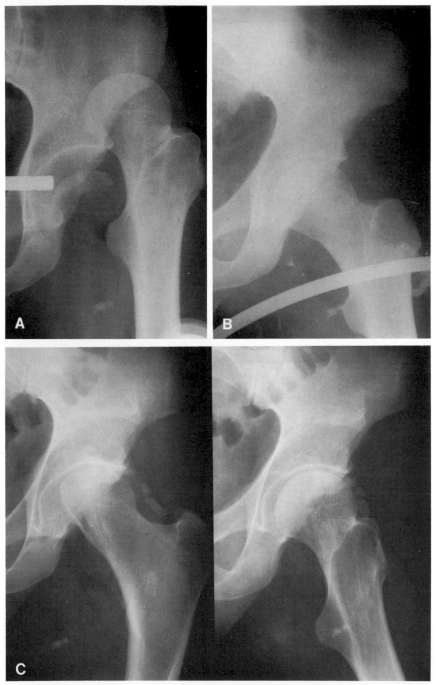

Fig. 3.40 J. M., a 29-year-old male, with type V dislocation, left, with supracondylar fracture, left femur. Primary open reduction was performed 8 days after injury. Follow-up 61 months later showed good result. *A*, roentgenogram, February 23, 1955. Note the fracture portion of the head in the acetabulum. Patient was unconscious and inoperable until 8 days after injury because of his poor condition. *B*, postreduction films, March 1, 1955. Approximately one-fourth of the medial portion of the femoral head was removed. There were loose fragments within the hip joint. *C*, roentgenograms (posterior-anterior and lateral), December 17, 1957. There is no avascular necrosis. Joint space is normal. Soft tissue calcification is minimal. Patient has good range of motion without pain, and is able to sit for hours without having to get up.

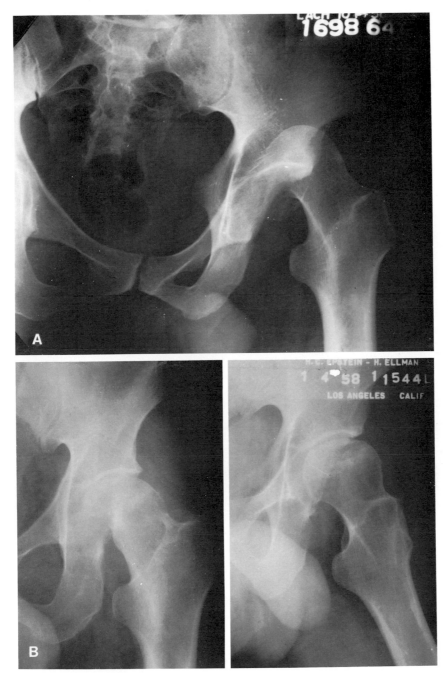

Fig. 3.41   This 34-year-old man, driving his automobile, struck a concrete wall, sustaining this type V posterior dislocation. A primary open reduction was done on the day of injury. The result at 15 months was rated good; at 18 months the result was poor, with avascular necrosis. *A,* roentgenogram on day of injury. The avulsed head fragment is faintly seen in the acetabulum. *B,* roentgenograms taken 18 months after surgery revealed avascular necrosis with depression of the weight-bearing portion of the head. One-fourth of the medial portion of the head was lying loose in the acetabulum. It was removed, as were many small loose fragments. There were numerous linear excoriations over the remaining portion of the head. The sciatic nerve was found stretched over the dislocated head, was thinned, attenuated, but not disrupted. There was no paralysis. Patient was having progressive pain in his hip and the hip was fused 30 months after injury.

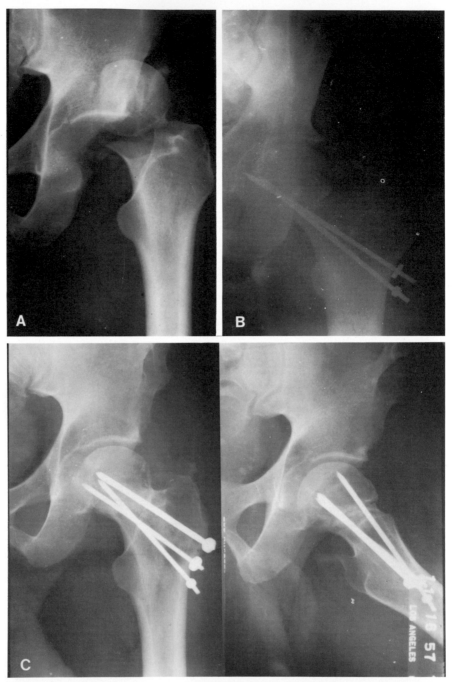

Fig. 3.42 P. E., a 39-year-old male, sustained this type V dislocation, left, with fracture of the femoral neck, when he was thrown out of a car in an auto accident. Primary open reduction with Moore pins and bone graft was performed. Follow-up at 18 months showed good result. *A*, roentgenogram June 30, 1956. Note the comminuted fragments about the head with the fracture through the femoral neck. *B*, roentgenogram July 2, 1956; primary open reduction 10 hours after injury, June 30, 1956. Several loose fragments were removed from the hip joint, which came off the femoral head. There was some attachment of the head to the neck by a small amount of capsule. This attachment was left intact after reduction was accomplished. Two Moore pins were inserted across the fracture site. *C*, roentgenogram, anterior and posterior, January 4, 1958. Bone graft from the ilium was placed across the neck of the femur into the head and an additional Moore nail was inserted August 2, 1956. The fracture of the neck was healed well. There is no evidence of avascular necrosis. There is minimal soft tissue calcification about the hip joint. Patient has good range of motion without pain, and has been working regularly for the past 6 months, doing light work. He is able to sit for hours without any aching, pain, or discomfort.

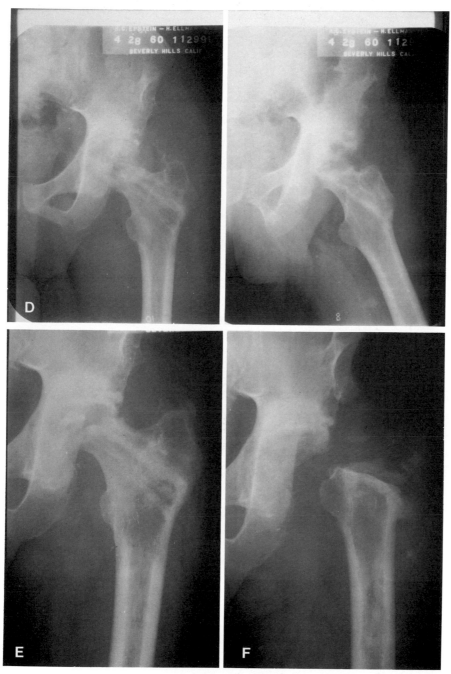

Fig. 3.42 *D,* three years after the original injury the patient was struck by a bale of rubber weighing 600 pounds. This caused one of the Moore pins to back out. Upon removal of this pin a localized infection of *Staphylococcus aureus,* coagulase-positive, was encountered. Roentgenogram reveals hip after all pins were removed. *E* and *F,* roentgenograms 5 years after dislocation. A girdlestone procedure was performed because of persistent pain and drainage. The patient gets along well with the use of a cane for support.

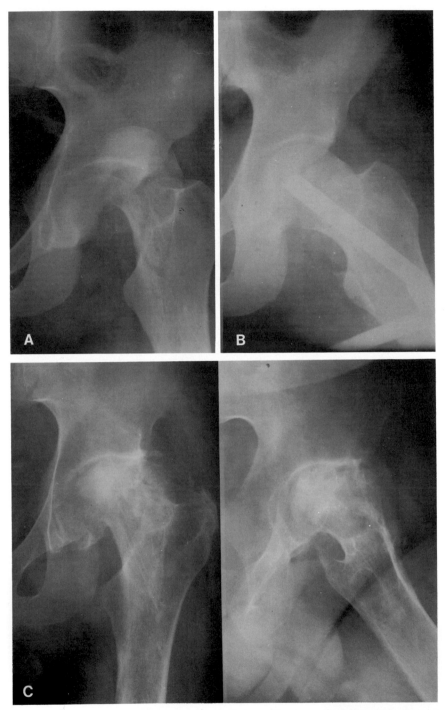

Fig. 3.43 A man, 26 years old, in an automobile collision, sustained a type V posterior dislocation of the left hip with a basal neck fracture, cerebral concussion, and fractures of the middle third of both femora. At follow-up 18 years later, after a primary open reduction, the result was poor. *A,* roentgenogram made on day of injury reveals the basal neck fracture and a large fragment of the femoral head lying in the acetabulum. Open reduction 6 days after injury consisted in removal of the head fragment and insertion of a Neufeld nail across the fracture site. *B,* The fractures are reduced and the Neufeld nail is in place. *C,* anteroposterior and lateral roentgenograms made 48 months after open reduction. At the time these roentgenograms were made the patient had moderate restriction of hip motion with soreness and aching of the hip after too much exercise. He was, however, able to bowl, swim, and perform his normal work in the electrical supply business. Eighteen years after his dislocation a total hip implant was contemplated because of severe hip pain.

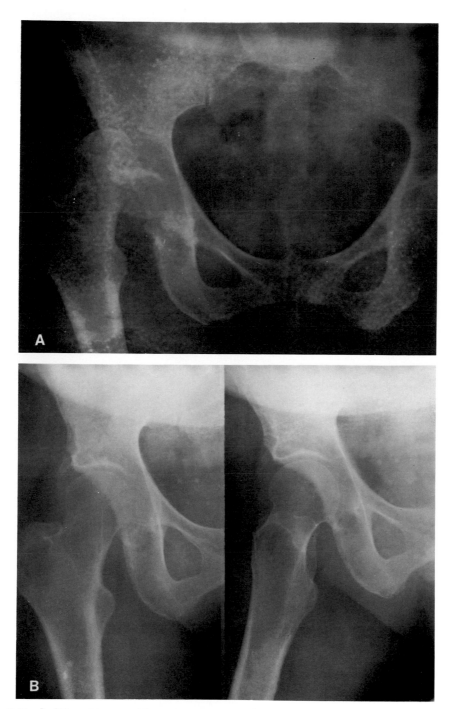

Fig. 3.44 L. W., a 64-year-old woman, passenger in an auto vs. auto accident, sustained a type V posterior fracture-dislocation of the right hip. A primary open reduction was performed on the day of injury through a posterior approach. The inferior third of the femoral head was discarded. Many small fragments were removed from the joint space. The result at follow-up 5 years later was good. Thirteen years after injury the result was rated poor with traumatic arthritis. *A*, roentgenogram reveals the posterior dislocation with a fracture of the inferior portion of the head. *B*, anteroposterior and lateral roentgenograms reveal normal joint space. There is minimal calcification over the superior portion of the head.

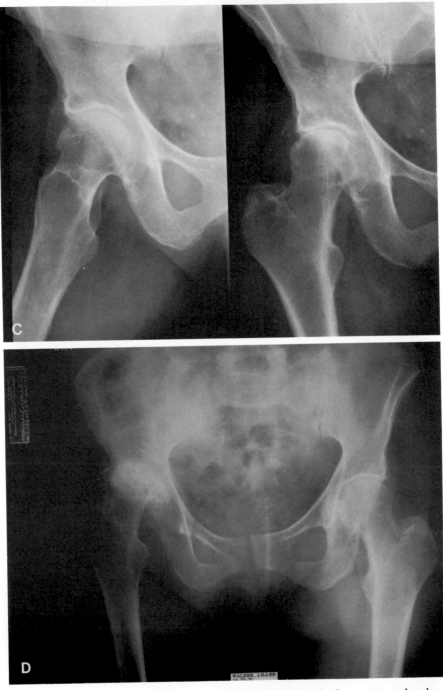

Fig. 3.44   *C,* the result 5 years after injury was good. Patient had no pain and only slight limitation of hip motion. Note beginning spur formation at the junction of the head and neck superiorly and minimal narrowing of the joint space, superiorly. *D,* thirteen years after injury there is traumatic arthritis of the right hip with moderate limitation of hip motion as well as severe pain. Symptoms started approximately 1 year prior to last examination after patient had a stroke involving the left lower extremity.

fragment of the femoral head and numerous fragments in the joint space were removed and the fracture of the neck was reduced and fixed with Moore pins. One month later, an iliac bone graft was inserted through the neck across the fracture site. The result was good (Fig. 3.42A-F). In the second, similar fragments were removed and the neck fracture was fixed with a Neufeld nail, but avascular necrosis developed and the result was poor 18 years after injury, when the patient had a total hip replacement because of severe hip pain (Fig. 3.43A-C). In the third, loose fragments were removed and the neck fracture was fixed with a Thompson "Z" nail 17 days after injury, but the hip became infected and a Girdlestone procedure was done. In the fourth, fragments were removed, the neck fracture was fixed with three Moore pins, and a Judet muscle-pedicle graft was done. At follow-up 15 months later the result was rated good, but at 24 months this was changed to poor.

With one exception the medial head fragment included approximately one-quarter to one-third of the femoral head in the type V hips with both good and unsatisfactory results. In the one exception the head fragment involved more than one-third of the head, including some of the weight-bearing portion.

Of the eight patients with good results one had a concurrent fracture of the femoral neck just mentioned. The other seven had head fragments removed which involved less than one-third of the head.

Of the two patients with fair results, one had numerous smaller fragments as well as the larger posterior medial fragment (5 × 3 × 0.5 cm) removed from the hip joint. The other patient previously mentioned had the muscle-pedicle graft.

Of the seven patients with unsatisfactory ratings, one was a 34-year-old man whose hip surgery was performed on the day of injury. Approximately one-third of the fractured medial femoral head was removed, as were the many loose fragments in the joint. The intact portion of the femoral head had linear excoriations on its articular surface. At 15 months the rating was good, but at 18 months it was poor because of moderate traumatic arthritis. The second patient was a 64-year-old woman who also had surgery on the day of injury. One-third of the femoral head was removed, as were many loose fragments in the joint; the result was good at 5 years but at 13 years traumatic arthritis had developed, the hip was painful and the patient had a poor result (Fig. 3.44A-D).

Four of the poor results were associated with avascular necrosis of the remaining portion of the head in two and in postoperative infections in two. In the last unsatisfactory case the acetabular labrum was torn off the posterior acetabulum and resutured. Two large defects in the femoral head were removed.

OVERALL INCIDENCE OF GOOD RESULTS

Primary open reduction yielded the highest proportion of good results after types II, III, and V fracture-dislocations, but after type IV lesions there was little

Table 3.4
Incidence of Good Results According to Type of Fracture-Dislocation and
Treatment

Type	Closed reduction (%)	Closed and open reduction (%)	Primary open reduction (%)
II	32	54	87
III	2	47	66
IV	15	31	40
V	0	33	47
Overall	15	41	60

difference between the results after open reduction and those after closed reduction followed by open reduction (Table 3.4). Closed reduction yielded a much lower proportion of good results after all four types of injury. The differences in incidence of good results were significant ($P < 0.05$) when primary open reduction was compared with the other methods used in types II, IV, and V lesions. In type II, however, the only significant difference was between primary open and closed reduction.

CHAPTER
4

ANTERIOR DISLOCATIONS IN ADULTS

Ninety-three anterior dislocations were analyzed in this series of 830 dislocations of the hip. This represents approximately 11% of all traumatic dislocations. There was adequate follow-up in 54 cases, with an average follow-up of 70.4 months. Anterior dislocations in children will be discussed in Chapter 5.

As in the case of posterior dislocations, an anterior dislocation demands early recognition as an emergency and prompt reduction. The typical attitude of an anterior dislocation is abduction and external rotation of the lower extremity (Figs. 1.28, 1.29, and 1.30).

There has been no reported extensive series of traumatic anterior dislocations from a large medical center. All previous studies have either been isolated case reports or have included anterior dislocations combined with posterior dislocations. Armstrong[3] reported on what appeared to be an obturator type dislocation with a fracture of the femoral head. Stewart and Milford[95] reported on 14 cases of anterior dislocations, designating them as anterior in six and obturator in eight. Results were excellent in three. Three had avascular necrosis and three had traumatic arthritis. Brav[9] mentioned 66 cases, with sufficient follow-up in 34. Excellent or good results occurred in 29, including one with avascular necrosis. Five had fair or poor results and two had avascular necrosis. Banks,[6] in reporting on aseptic necrosis of the femoral head following traumatic dislocation of the hip, reported six obturator dislocations. Stuck and Vaughn[98] reported two anterior and two obturator dislocations in 44 total dislocations. Funsten[2] et al.[132] had two obturator dislocations in a total of 20 cases. Hamada[42] reported on seven cases of unreduced anterior dislocations of the hip, three fresh and four old unreduced. Aggarwal and Singh[1] also reported on seven unreduced cases; one a bilateral dislocation. Others who reported anterior dislocations, all with complications, are Hampson,[44] Katznelson,[56] Henderson,[49] Dingley,[18] and Helal et al.[48]

MECHANISM OF INJURY

Most of the anterior dislocated hips in this series were due to automobile accidents (Table 1.6). Either the knee struck the dashboard with the thighs abducted or the patient was thrown out of the vehicle. Seatbelts would be important in preventing the forward thrust, or ejection, in many of these cases. One patient, however, dislocated her hip when she, as well as the seatbelt and the seat, were thrown out of the car.

Anterior dislocations of the hip may result from falls or crushing injuries received on the back of the pelvis with the hip in a position of abduction. In an unusual case reported by Aggarwal and Singh,[1] the patient was stooping and a blow from a falling object struck the lower part of the back, forcing the lower limb into flexion, abduction, and external rotation causing an obturator dislocation.

An anterior dislocation can be sustained with what appears to be a trivial injury such as one which occurred when a wave overturned a patient while he was swimming (Fig. 1.16). It has also occurred when a patient falls downstairs, falls out of bed, or trips while walking. The apparent ease with which some anterior dislocations can occur does not usually happen in posterior dislocations, which are generally sustained by more violent trauma.

THEORY AS TO THE PRODUCTIVITY OF ANTERIOR DISLOCATIONS OF THE HIP

The most important factor in producing an anterior dislocation is forcible abduction. The neck or trochanter impinges upon the rim of the acetabulum and

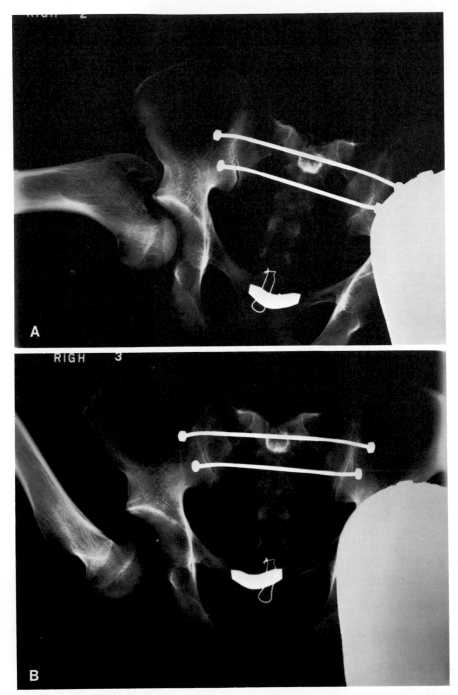

Fig. 4.1 *A,* theory as to production of an anterior dislocations. The most important factor is forcible abduction; neck or trochanter impinges upon rim of acetabulum and head of femur is levered out of its socket and through anterior capsule. *B,* external rotation tends to force the head forward through the capsule. Compression or fracture of the femoral head may occur when the head impinges on the superior anterior acetabular lip or on the inferior lip when the head moves downward.

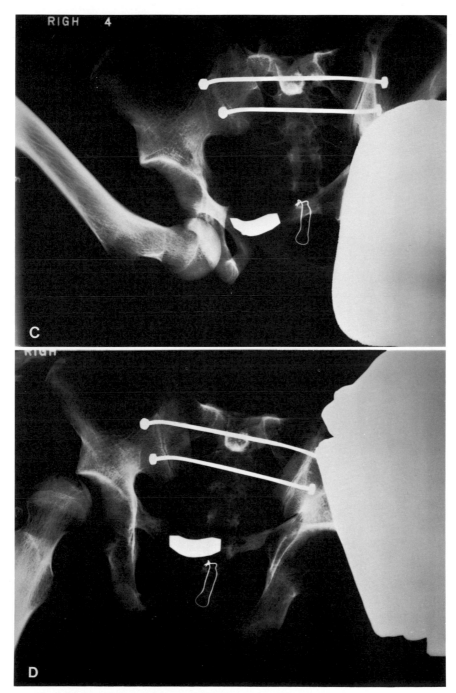

Fig. 4.1 *C,* if the hip is in a position of flexion an obturator dislocation may occur. *D,* with extension of the hip, the head tends to move upward to the public region:

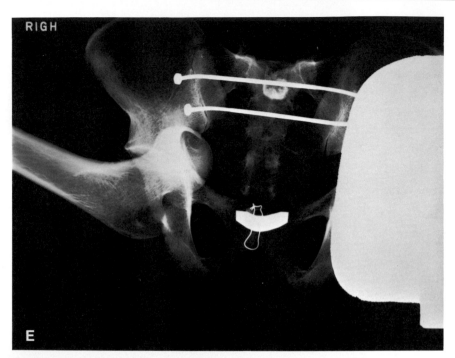

Fig. 4.1 *E,* or the femoral head may cross over the pubic area anteriorly.

Table 4.1
Anterior Dislocations

A. Pubic (superior)
  1. With no fracture (simple)
  2. With fracture of head of femur
  3. With fracture of acetabulum
B. Obturator (inferior)
  1. With no fracture (simple)
  2. With fracture of head of femur
  3. With fracture of acetabulum

the head of the femur is levered out of its socket and through the capsule (Fig. 4.1*A–E*). External rotation tends to force the head forward through the capsule. Compression of the femoral head may occur when the head impinges on the inferior lip of the acetabulum as the head moves downward. If the hip is in a position of flexion, an obturator dislocation occurs; if the hip is extended the head tends to move upward to the pubic area or cross over the pubic area anteriorly.

CLASSIFICATION

The anterior dislocations were divided into pubic and obturator types (Table 4.1). There were 84 obturator dislocations (Fig. 4.2), including a scrotal type (Fig. 4.3*A–E*) and nine pubic dislocations (Fig. 4.4*A, B*). Seven of the total 93 dislocations were bilateral (Figs. 4.5; 4.6*A–C*; 4.7*A–C*; 4.8*A–C*; 4.9*A–C*), with an anterior on one side and a posterior on the other. There was also a bilateral anterior dislocation (Fig. 4.9*A, B*). Compression of the femoral head (Fig. 4.10*A–E*) or a fracture of the femoral head or trochanter occurred in eleven cases (Figs.

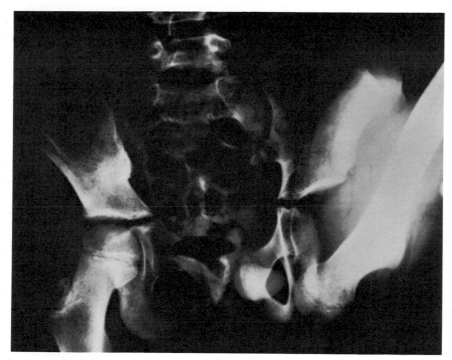

Fig. 4.2   Anterior (obturator) dislocation, left hip.

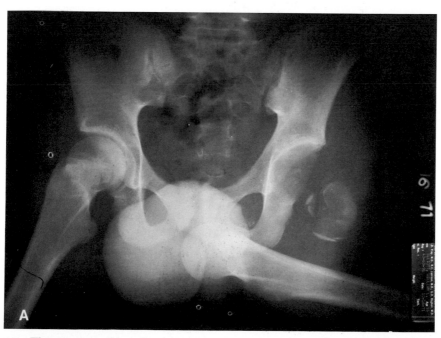

Fig. 4.3   This 16-year-old male sustained this anterior dislocation of the left hip with displacement into the scrotal area in a motorcycle accident. The result after 15 months is fair with avascular necrosis. (Figs. 4.3A–E, courtesy of George J. Wiesseman, M.D., San Bernardino.) A, note the dislocation of the left hip lying in the region of the scrotum with avulsion of the greater trochanter.

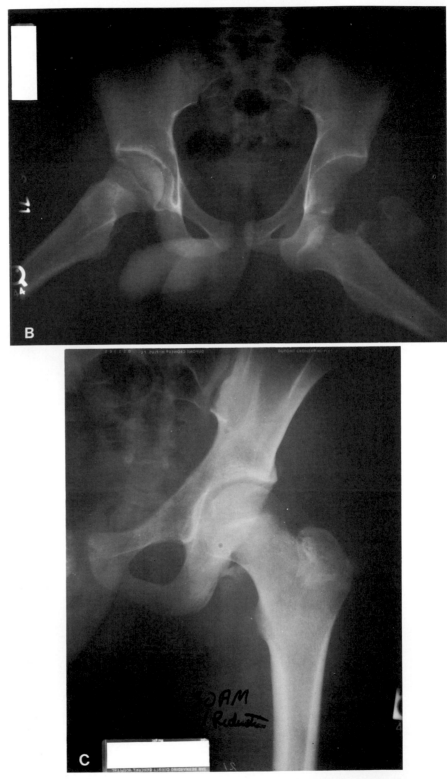

Fig. 4.3 *B,* after reduction under a general anesthesia the dislocation appears to be an obturator type. *C,* at a second attempt the hip was reduced and the greater trochanter appears to be reattached. Because of instability it was necessary to secure the trochanter with two screws.

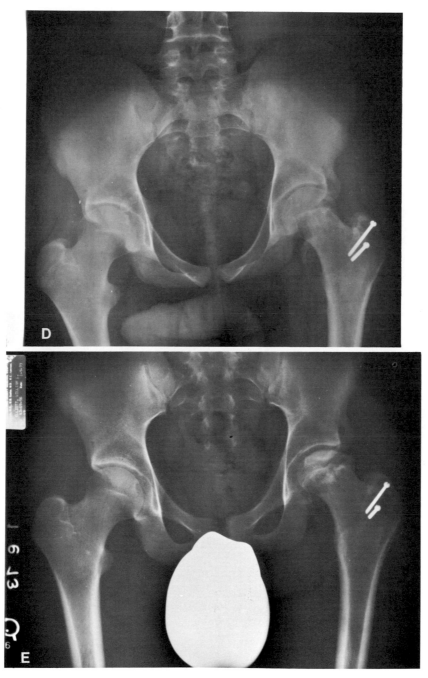

Fig. 4.3 *D*, eleven months after reduction, the left hip joint appears normal and the greater trochanter has fused to the shaft of the femur. *E*, fifteen months after injury there is avascular necrosis of the femoral head. A derotational osteotomy was performed but the results are unknown.

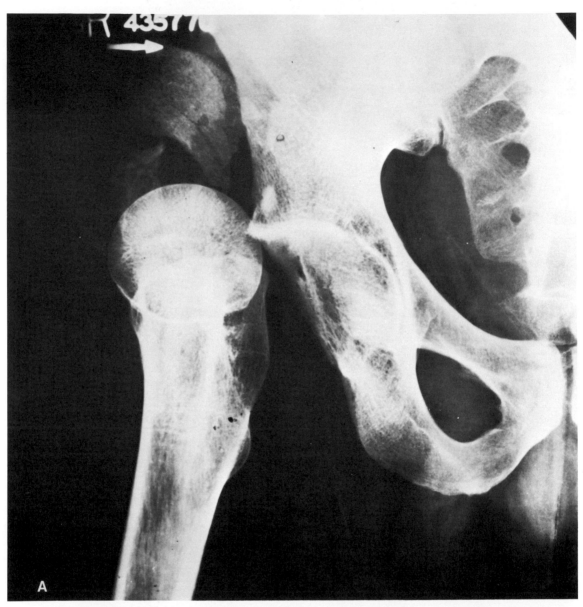

Fig. 4.4 *A,* anterior dislocation (pubic) with fracture of ilium. A 28-year-old male was swimming in ocean when wave overturned him. Hip was easily reduced under general anesthesia by flexion of hip, direct traction in line with femur and internal rotation.

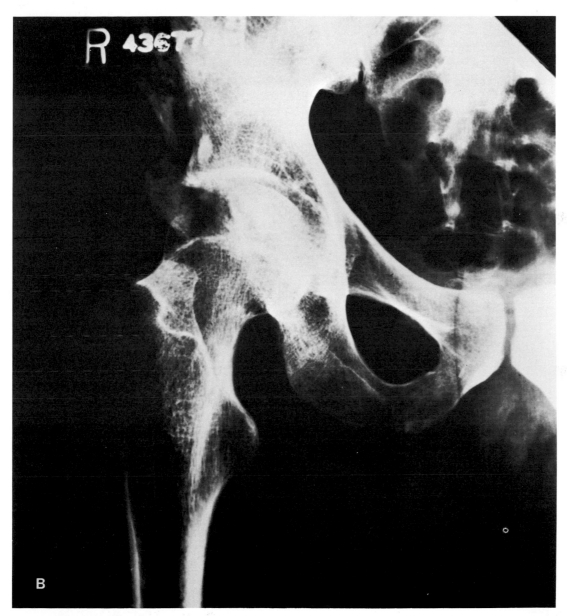

Fig. 4.4 *B,* after closed reduction. Result unknown because of insufficient follow-up.

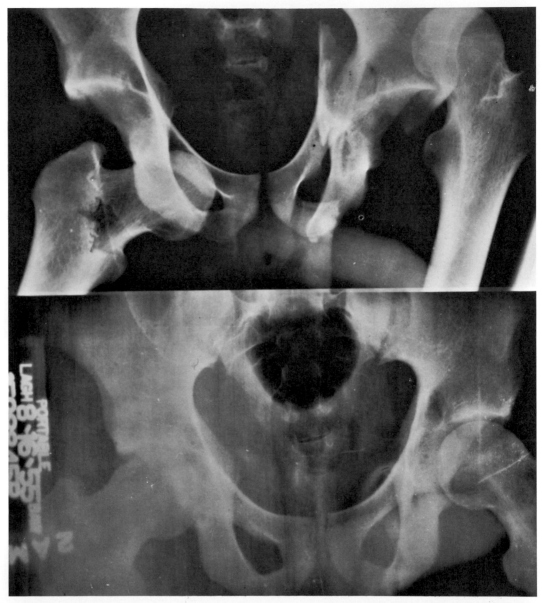

Fig. 4.5   This is a bilateral anterior dislocation on the right and a type IV posterior dislocation on the left in a 17-year-old male involved in an automobile accident. Both dislocations were reduced easily on the day of injury under general anesthesia. The patient died of multiple injuries 24 hours later. (From Epstein, H. C.: Traumatic anterior and simple posterior dislocations of the hip in adults and children. In *The American Academy of Orthopaedic Surgeons: Instructional Course Lectures*, vol. 22. The C. V. Mosby Co., St. Louis, 1973. Reproduced with permission.)

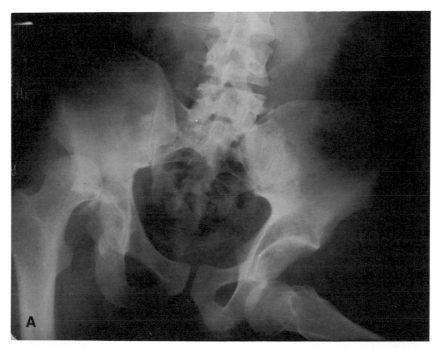

Fig. 4.6 A 26-year-old male was involved in a head-on collision, sustaining this bilateral dislocation, a type IV on the right side and an obturator dislocation on the left. Both dislocations were reduced without difficulty on the day of injury under general anesthesia. The posterior dislocation was opened 12 days after injury with removal of many loose fragments from the hip joint. No attempt was made to approximate the fracture through the acetabular floor. The result 13 months after injury was excellent for the anterior dislocation and fair for the posterior injury. A, note the multiple fragments about the hip joint on the right side and the obturator dislocation on the left.

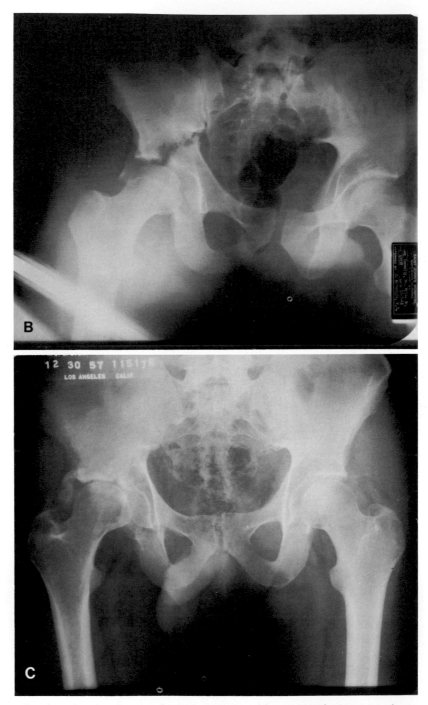

Fig. 4.6 *B,* after closed reduction the right hip resembles a central protrusion fracture. The left hip shows a normal reduction. *C,* thirteen months after open reduction of the right hip the joint space appears narrowed and the posterior rim fragment is displaced laterally. The fracture through the floor of the acetabulum was healed. The left hip is normal.

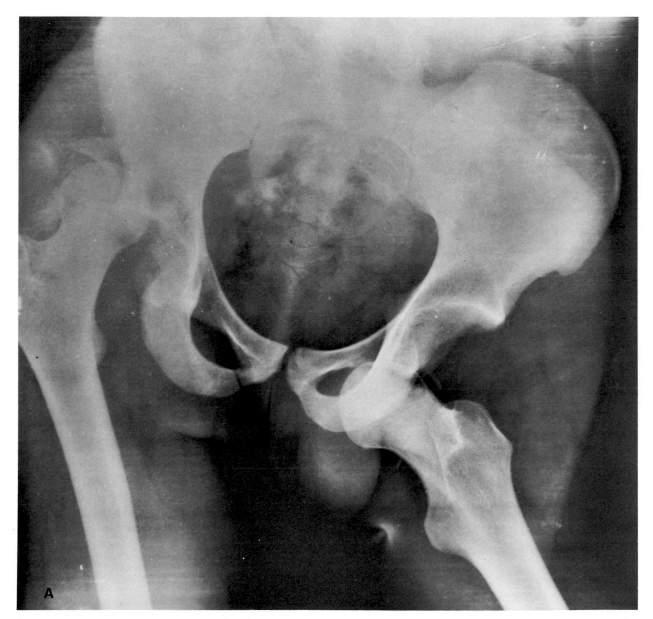

Fig. 4.7   W. H., a 22-year-old male injured in an automobile vs. wall accident. *A*, the patient sustained bilateral dislocation of the hip, anterior on the left and posterior type III on the right, with a fair result on the left side.

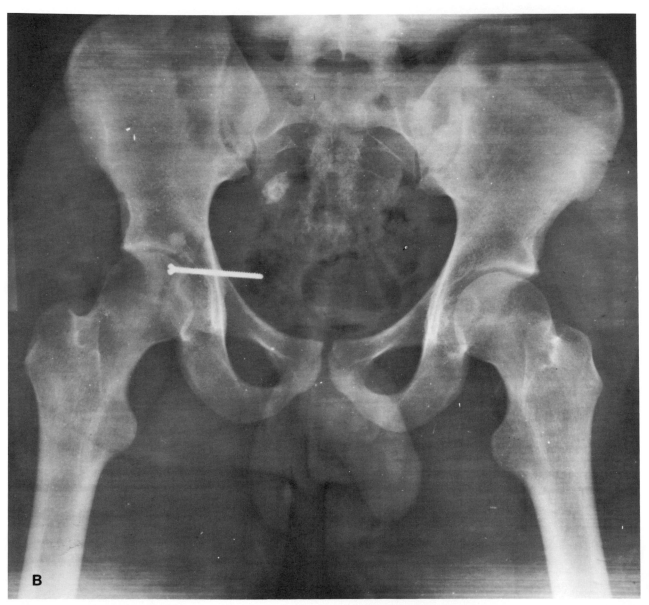

Fig. 4.7 *B*, a primary open reduction was performed on the posterior dislocation of the right hip and a closed reduction under general anesthesia on the left. He was in traction for 6 weeks and then started weight-bearing.

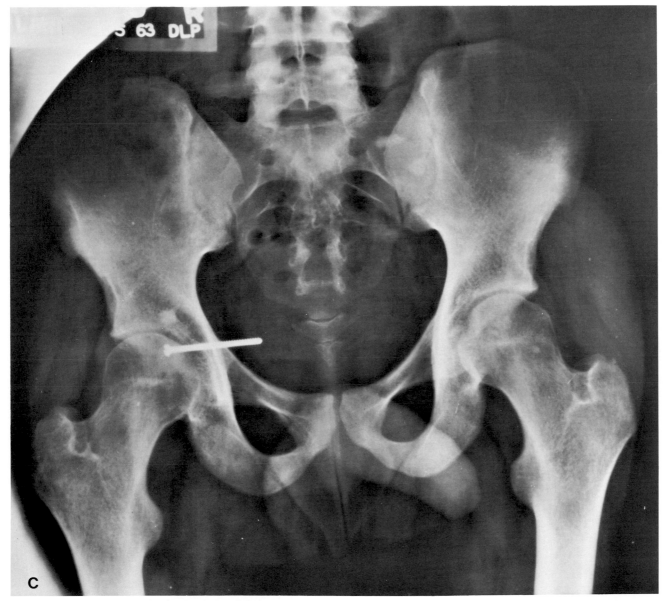

Fig. 4.7 C, six months after injury there is flattening of the lateral portion of the femoral head of the left hip with minimal narrowing of the joint space. The patient was lost to follow-up after 6 months and the result of the right hip is unknown.

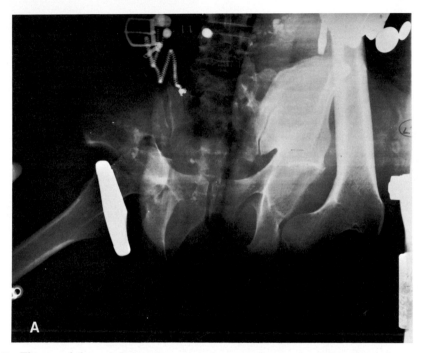

Fig. 4.8 This is a bilateral dislocation; central protrusion on the right side and an anterior obturator dislocation on the left with a complete sciatic paralysis. This young man was run over twice by his wife in an attempt to kill him. (This case was not used in the statistics and was sent to me by Charles A. Owen, M.D.) *A*, note the anterior dislocation (left) which is at right angle to the acetabulum. The right hip reveals a central protrusion fracture involving a portion of the acetabular dome and the posterior column.

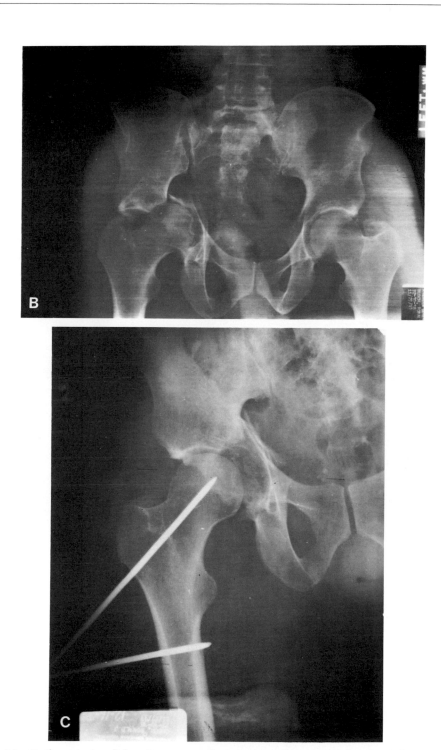

Fig. 4.8 *B,* the anterior dislocation was easily reduced under general anesthesia by traction. *C,* the central protrusion fracture was reduced by traction with pins in the neck and shaft of the femur just below the lesser trochanter. The result is not known because of insufficient follow-up.

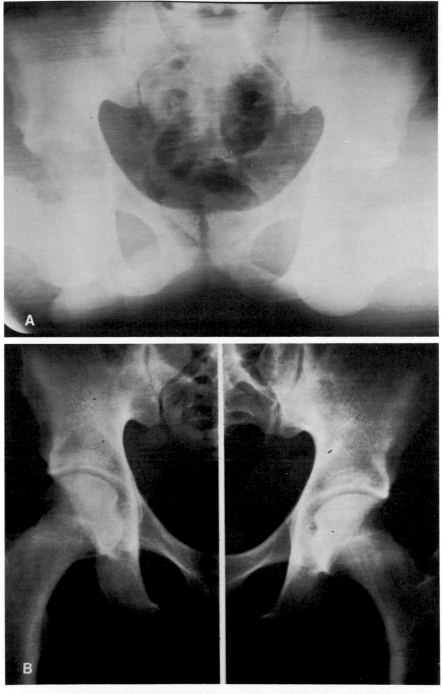

Fig. 4.9 This is a 20-year-old male with a bilateral anterior dislocation of both hips sustained in auto accident as a passenger. Both hips were widely abducted at the time of accident. No seatbelt was worn. *A,* note obturator dislocations both hips. *B,* hip dislocations were reduced easily under general anesthesia on day of injury. (This case sent to me courtesy of Stanford Noel, M.D.; not used in the statistics because of insufficient follow-up.)

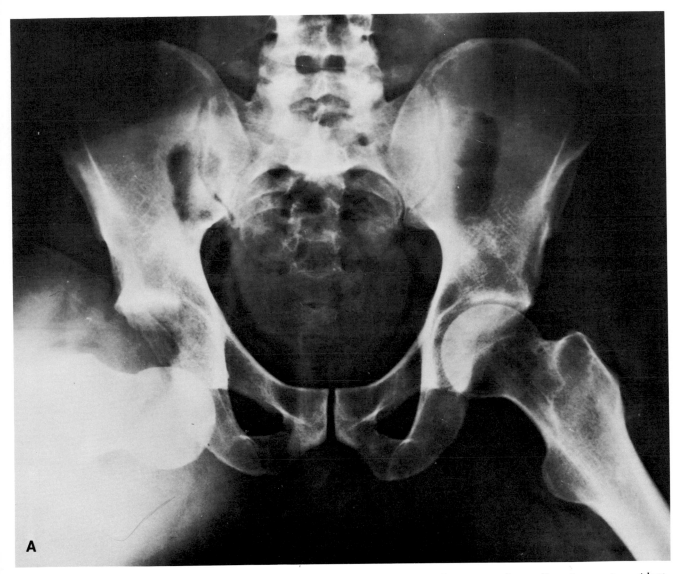

A

Fig. 4.10 Compression of the femoral head. *A*, a 32-year-old male passenger was thrown out of a small car in an auto accident. This is an obturator dislocation.

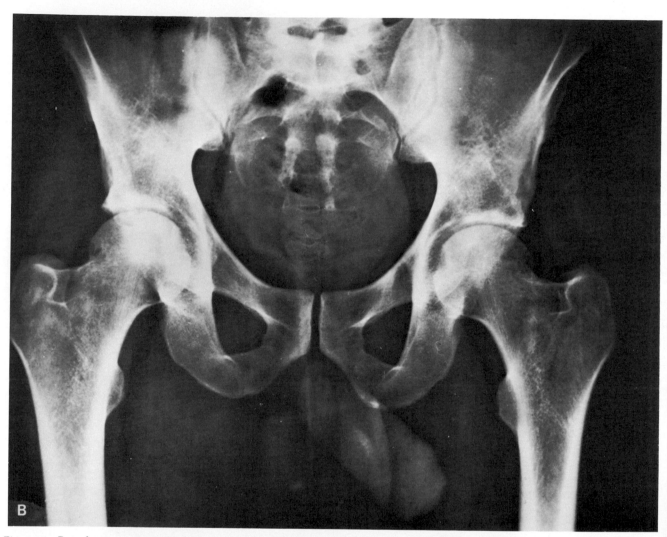

Fig. 4.10 *B,* reduction was performed on the day of injury. Note defect in femoral head.

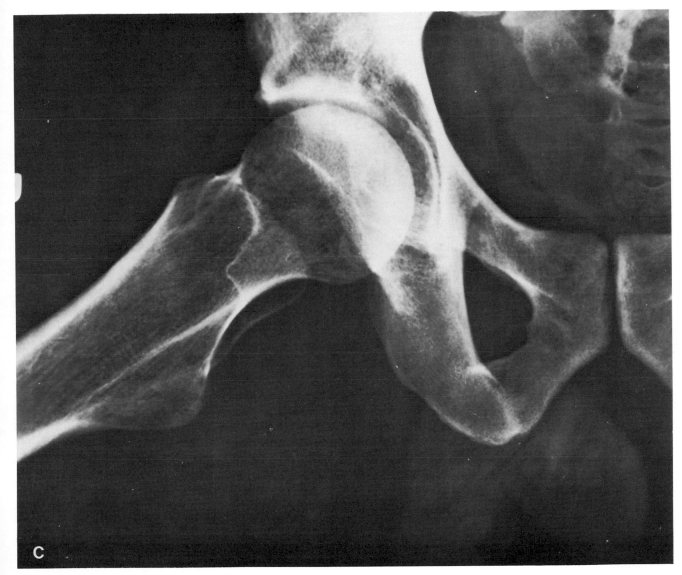

Fig. 4.10 C, lateral view showing defect in head of femur. Patient was transferred to private care.

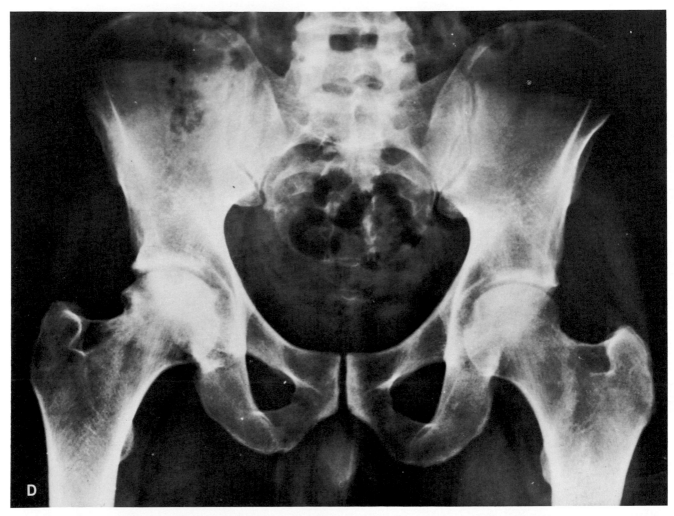

Fig. 4.10 *D,* at 2½ years after injury, anteroposterior roentgenograms reveal traumatic arthritis, although it looks like avascular necrosis. There are areas of increased and decreased densities in femoral head, with narrowing of joint space and spur formation on the neck, superiorly and inferiorly.

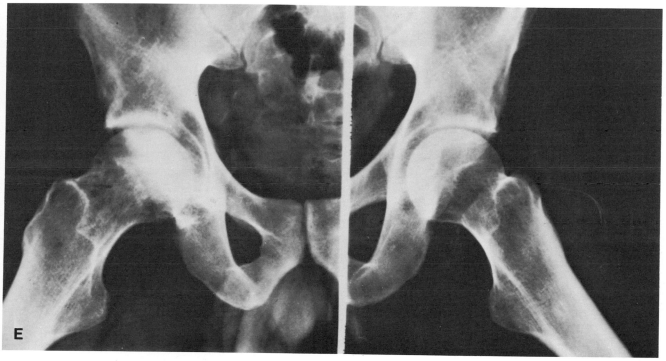

Fig. 410 *E,* lateral roentgenogram, comparing abnormal with normal hip. Patient has 1½ inches of atrophy of right thigh, moderate limitation of hip motion, and intermittent hip pain. Result is fair.

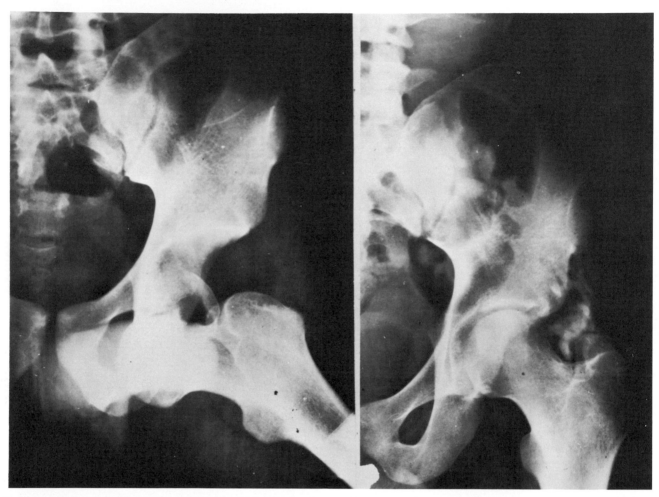

Fig. 4.11   A 21-year-old male in an auto vs. highway divider accident sustained anterior dislocation with fracture of femoral head. A primary open reduction through anterior approach was performed on the day of injury. A large, loose fragment of bone was off the femoral head and lying in the joint, but it did not involve too much of the weight-bearing portion of the head. Russell traction was applied for 5 weeks, weight-bearing was started in 2 months. Although there was calcification about the capsule, the result in 13 months was considered good.

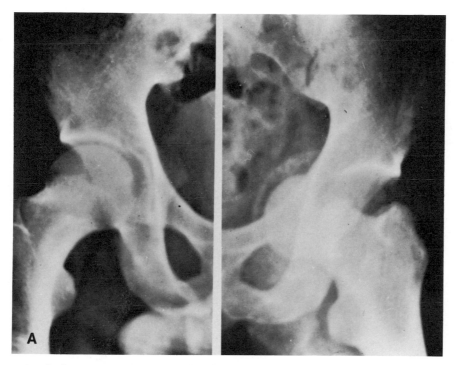

Fig. 4.12 *A,* this 24-year-old man sustained this anterior dislocation (pubic) in auto vs. tree accident. There was a cerebral contusion and spastic paralysis. Roentgenograms 3½ weeks later revealed dislocation.

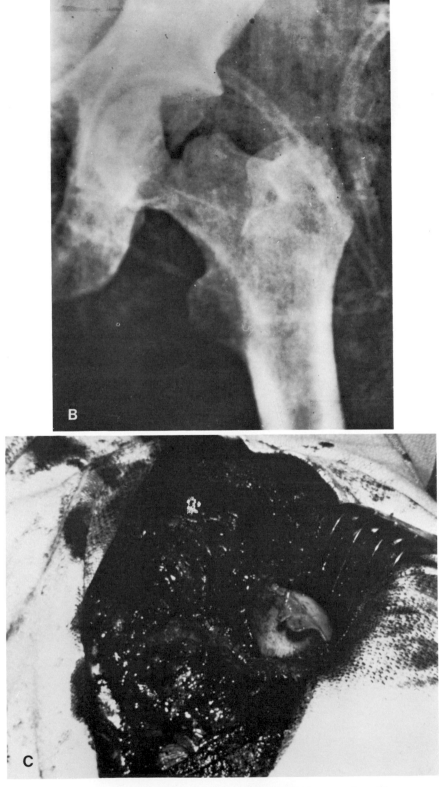

Fig. 4.12 *B,* anteroposterior roentgenogram after surgery. Note large wedge of bone removed from femoral head. *C,* at surgery the head of the femur was wedged against brim of pubic bone. Note large defect in superior lateral portion of head.

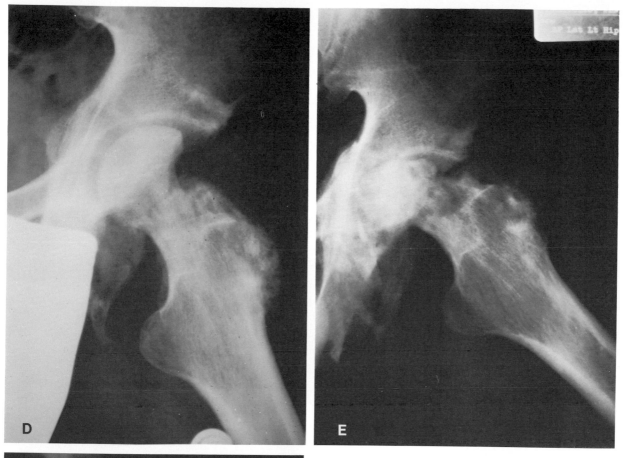

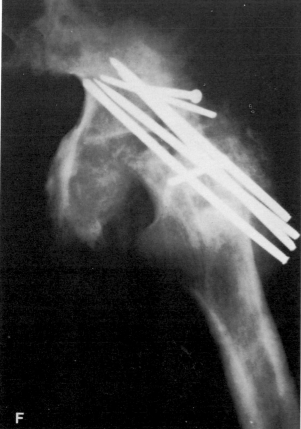

Fig. 4.12 *D* and *E,* roentgenograms showing progressive degenerative changes in the left hip 6 and 10 months after open reduction. *F,* fusion of hip 15 months after injury.

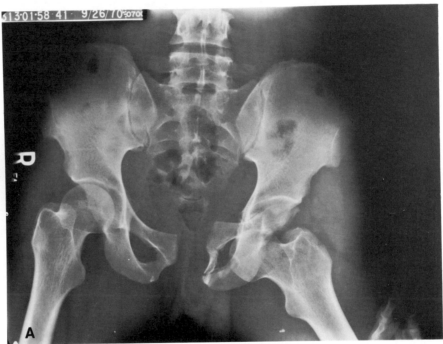

Fig. 4.13 *A,* a 37-year-old man, riding a motorcycle which collided with an automobile, sustained this anterior obturator dislocation of the left hip with fractures of the left pubic bone and acetabulum. He also had multiple injuries including a complete dislocation of cervical II on cervical I, a cardiac contusion, bilateral pneumothorax, and a compound, comminuted fracture of the left tibia and fibula. Closed reduction of the dislocated hip was unsuccessful on day of injury.

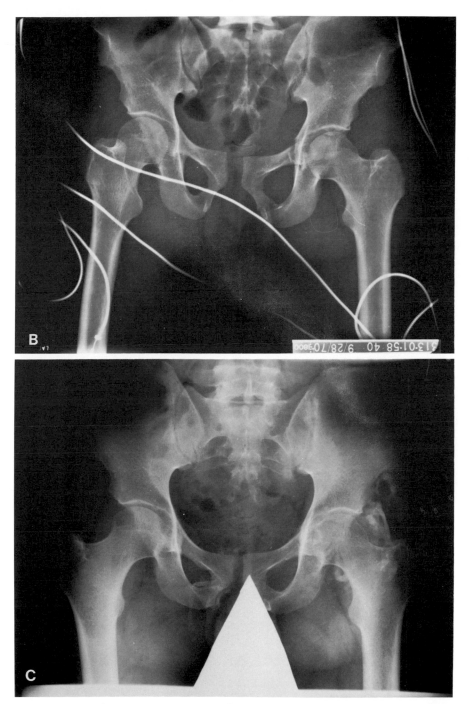

Fig. 4.13 *B*, open reduction (anterior approach) was performed 3 weeks after injury. Hip was irreducible because a segment of the pubic bone jutted into the acetabulum with the femoral head lying anterior to this fracture. *C*, at 30 months after injury there is moderate myositis ossificans with some flattening of the lateral portion of the femoral head. The joint space appears normal. There is no evidence of avascular necrosis. Patient uses a cane because of stiffness and feeling of pressure in the left hip. The case is rated fair. Prognosis is guarded as to traumatic arthritis.

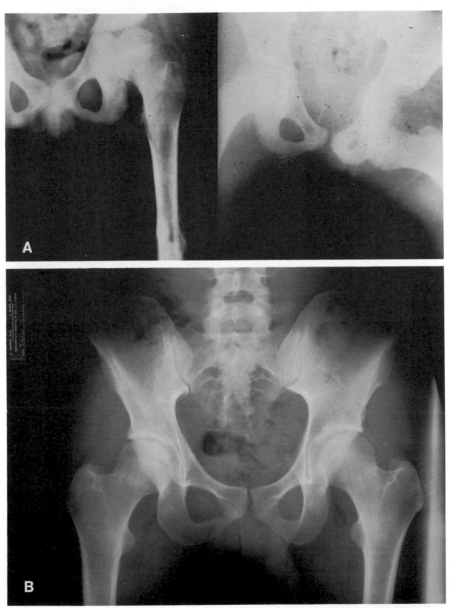

Fig. 4.14 *A,* An anterior dislocation of the left hip and an ipsilateral fracture of the femur in a 12-year-old boy, with an excellent result 13 years later. He was struck by an automobile, fracturing the left femur. The dislocated hip was recognized when a roentgenogram of the pelvis was ordered by an orthopaedic resident. The dislocated hip was reduced by inserting a tibial pin and then applying fraction while patient was under general anesthesia. The hip and femur were placed in balanced traction for 3 months, then weight-bearing gradually started. *B,* at 13 years after injury the result is still excellent with normal roentgenogram and normal motion of the hip. The femur is well healed with excellent alignment.

4.11; 4.12*A–F*). Seven of the dislocations had concurrent fractures of the acetabulum (4.13*A–C*). Ipsilateral fracture of the femur occurred in two of the dislocations, both recognized at the time of injury (Fig. 4.14*A, B*), and in nine of the dislocations there were multiple injuries.

RESULTS

The results in the 54 anterior dislocations with adequate follow-up were as follows (Table 4.2). Seventeen had excellent and 21 good results (70%) (Figs. 4.15*A–C*; 4.15*A, B*). Eleven had fair and five poor results (30%). All the satisfactory results were in obturator dislocations, with one sustaining a fracture of the femoral head with subsequent primary open reduction and the other with an open procedure following an unsuccessful attempt at closed reduction.

In the case with the fracture of the femoral head (Fig. 4.11), the surgery was performed through an anterior approach and a large fragment of bone was found loose in the hip joint. The fragment came off the superior-anterior portion of the femoral head (as contrasted with type V posterior dislocations in which the head fragment is avulsed off the posterior-medial portion of the femoral head) and did not involve too much of the weight-bearing portion of the head. The fragment was removed.

The second case (Fig. 4.17*A, B*) was a bilateral dislocation in a 49-year-old passenger in an automobile accident. There were three unsuccessful attempts at reduction of the anterior dislocation. An open reduction was performed on the day of injury. This revealed the tendon of the iliopsoas to be stretched anteriorly across the neck of the femur and held tightly in position. It was possible to slip the iliopsoas tendon under the head of the femur with traction and complete flexion of the hip and the hip then reduced easily. Katznelson[56] reported a similar case, in which the femoral head had been driven through the iliopsoas muscle, preventing closed reduction.

All obturator dislocations with excellent or good results were reduced in under 24 hours on the first attempt except for the two cases mentioned previously. Two had ipsilateral femoral fractures recognized at the time of injury. In the fair or poor results, eleven of the dislocations all reduced in under 24 hours had either a fracture of the femoral head or trochanter or a compression of the femoral head or were reduced later than 24 hours after injury.

In the two obturator dislocations with avascular necrosis, one was a simple dislocation and in the other case the greater trochanter was avulsed. In the simple dislocation (Fig. 1.43), a 25-year-old male, while on board a fishing boat, had a hopper weighing ½ ton fall on him, pinning him to the floor. The hip was not reduced until at least 18 hours later when the boat landed in Lima, Peru. Weight-bearing was started 30 days after traction. The patient stated he experienced

Table 4.2
Results in 54 Anterior Dislocations of the Hip in Adults[a]

Excellent	Good	Fair	Poor	Total	Percentage of excellent-good results
17	21	11	5	54	70

[a] Average follow-up, 70.4 months.

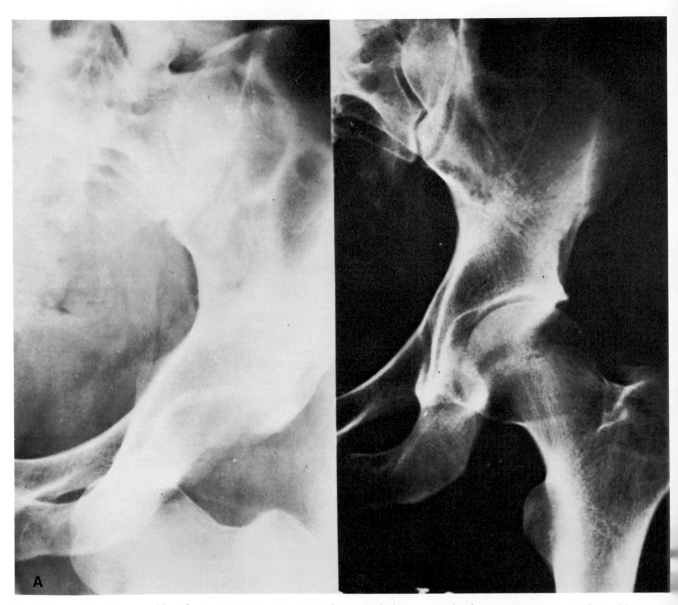

Fig. 4.15   *A,* this 23-year-old male, passenger in an auto without seatbelt, was involved in auto vs. auto accident. Obturator dislocation was reduced on the day of the accident. He was in traction for 6 weeks; discarded crutches by the 4th week.

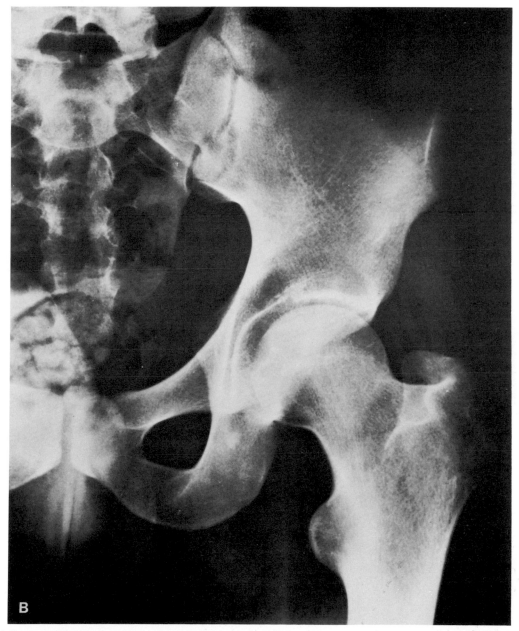

Fig. 4.15 *B,* follow-up films 3 years later, with excellent result. Traction for 5 weeks was followed by weight-bearing. Range of hip motion is normal, without complaints.

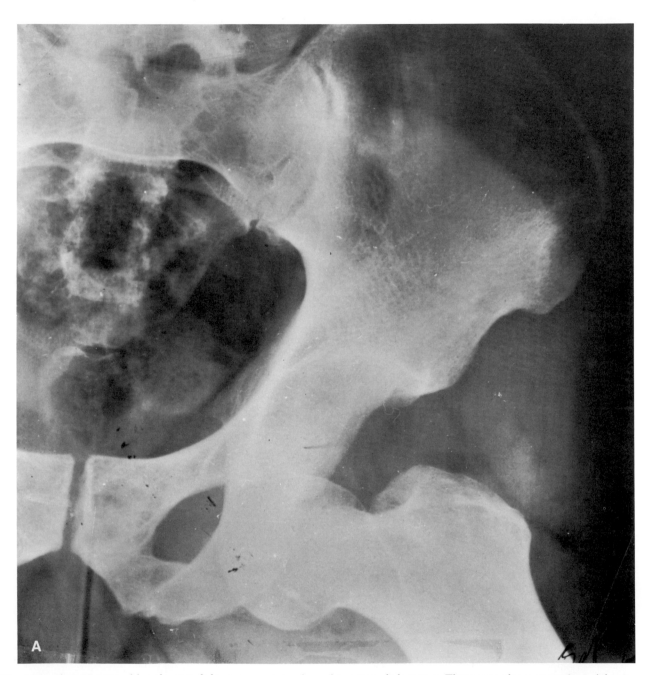

Fig. 4.16 *A,* a 28-year-old male, struck by auto, sustained an obturation dislocation. There was also a contralateral fracture of the extremity.

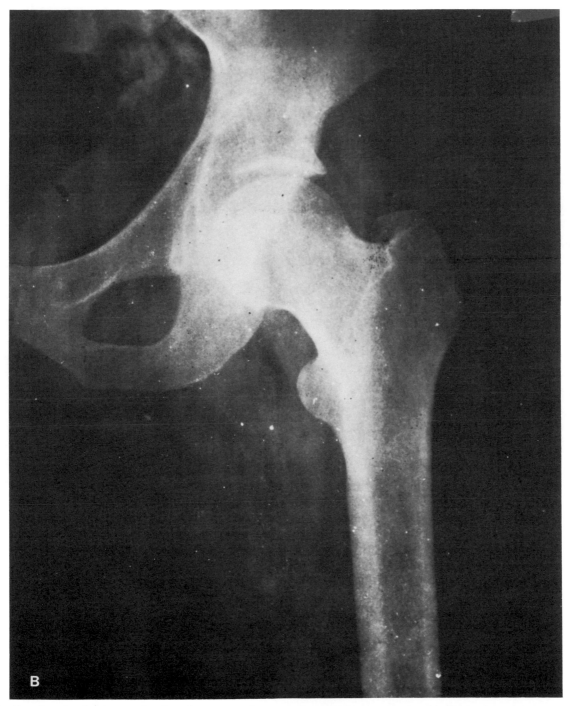

Fig. 4.16 *B,* a closed reduction on the day of injury, under general anesthesia, was successful. Skeletal traction was applied for 12 days, followed by bed rest for 3 weeks, and then weight-bearing. Results 5 years later were good. Roentgenograms were normal, but patient had minimal restrictions on internal and external rotation of hip.

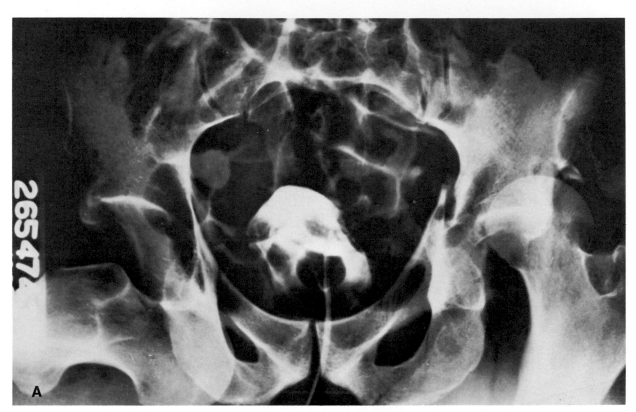

Fig. 4.17   *A,* a 48-year-old male, passenger in an auto collision, sustained a bilateral dislocation, with an anterior on the right and posterior on the left. At 2 years the result was rated good on both hips. There were three unsuccessful attempts at closed reduction of the anterior dislocation, which was then opened on the day of injury. The iliopsoas tendon was found to be wrapped around the base of the neck, preventing closed reduction. Primary open reduction was performed for the left hip dislocation, with removal of fragments from the hip joint. No attempt was made to transfix the acetabular floor fracture.

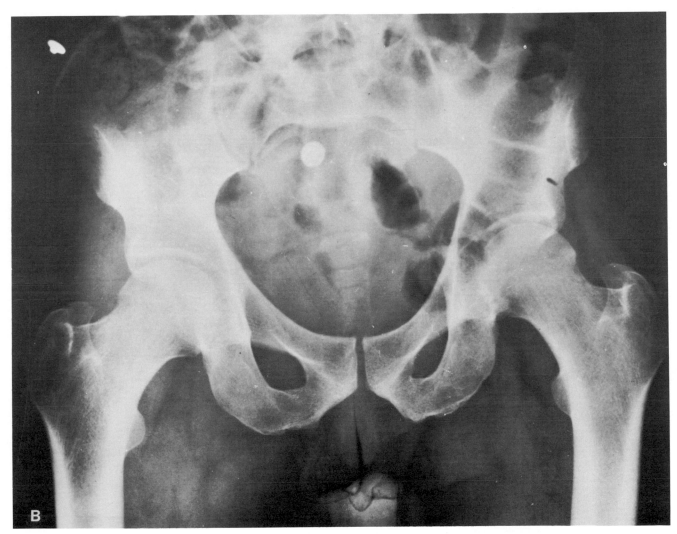

Fig. 4.17 *B,* patient was kept in traction for 2 months, and started weightbearing in 3 months. There was good motion of both hips. (From Epstein, H. C.: Traumatic anterior and simple posterior dislocations of the hip in adults and children. In *The American Academy of Orthopaedic Surgeons: Instructional Course Lectures,* vol. 22. The C. V. Mosby Co., St. Louis, 1973. Reproduced with permission.)

constant hip pain since weight-bearing. Avascular necrosis was evident on roent-genograms 8 months after reduction.

The second case of avascular necrosis (Fig. 4.3A–E) occurred in a 16-year-old male who was involved in a motorcycle accident. The greater trochanter was avulsed. The dislocation was first a scrotal dislocation, pulled into the obturator position and then reduced. The greater trochanter was fixed with two screws 2 days after the closed reduction. Avascular necrosis was evident 16 months after reduction.

In one of the two cases with myositis ossificans, there was a bilateral dislocation, anterior on one side and posterior on the other. Both hips developed this condition (Fig. 3.3). In the second case the obturator dislocation with a fracture of the acetabulum was irreducible by closed methods and because of multiple injuries the open procedure was delayed three and a half weeks (Fig. 4.12).

ROENTGENOGRAPHIC JOINT CHANGES

There were 16 fair or poor results in the 54 dislocations with sufficient follow-up (Table 4.3). In the miscellaneous group one was rated fair clinically but the roentgenogram was normal; in another, a pubic dislocation with an acetabular fracture, the hip redislocated in this 79-year-old woman but no attempt was made to relocate it; in the other case, also a pubic type in an 81-year-old woman, the neck of the femur was fractured during the attempt at closed reduction (Fig. 4.18A, B).

Nine of the hips with traumatic arthritis were obturator types with compression of the femoral head. This compression or fracture of the superior anterior portion of the femoral head occurs when the head impinges on the inferior lip of the acetabulum as the head moves downward when it is levered out of the acetabular socket through the capsule with the hip in flexion (Fig. 4.1).

In the obturator dislocation in which the greater trochanter is avulsed the mechanism was probably impingement on the superior lip of the acetabulum as the femoral head was levered out. A similar type of injury was described by Katznelson.[56]

Five dislocations with unsatisfactory results were of the pubic type with fracture of the femoral head, acetabulum, or pubic bone. In one of these, a 24-year-old male sustained a spastic paralysis (Fig. 4.12A–F) following a cerebral concussion. The dislocation was not recognized for 3½ weeks when roentgeno-grams were taken of the pelvis. At surgery the head and neck were wedged against the superior brim of the acetabulum. Approximately one-half of the femoral head was broken off into fragments and had to be removed 6 months after injury. Because of severe hip pain an arthrodesis was performed.

Table 4.3
Roentgenographic Joint Changes in 16 Anterior Dislocations in Adults with Fair or Poor Results

	Avascular necrosis	Traumatic arthritis	Myositis ossificans	Miscellaneous	Total
Total	2	9	2	3[a]	16
Percentage	4%	17%	4%	6%	

[a] One hip redislocated into posterior dislocation (not reduced); one hip neck of femur fractured in attempt at closed reduction; and one hip was fair clinical, x-rays normal.

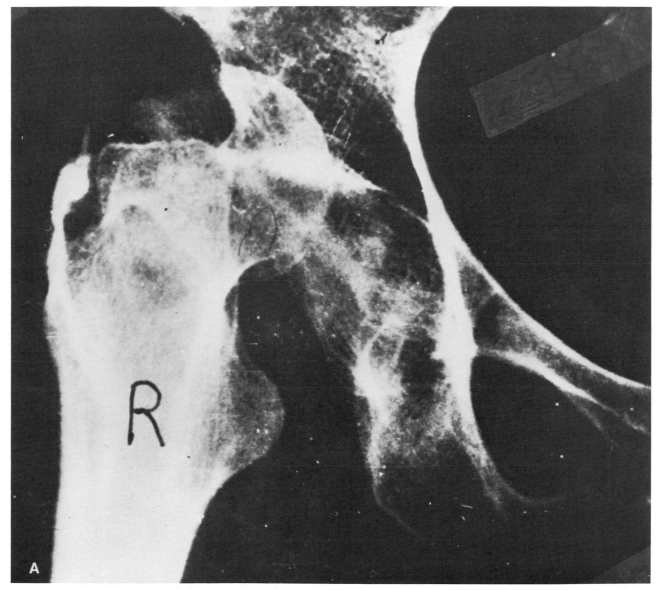

Fig. 4.18 *A,* this pubic anterior dislocation occurred in an 81-year-old woman who fell while crossing a street. Femoral head is anterior to superior rim of acetabulum. Courtesy of Fred Polesky, M.D.)

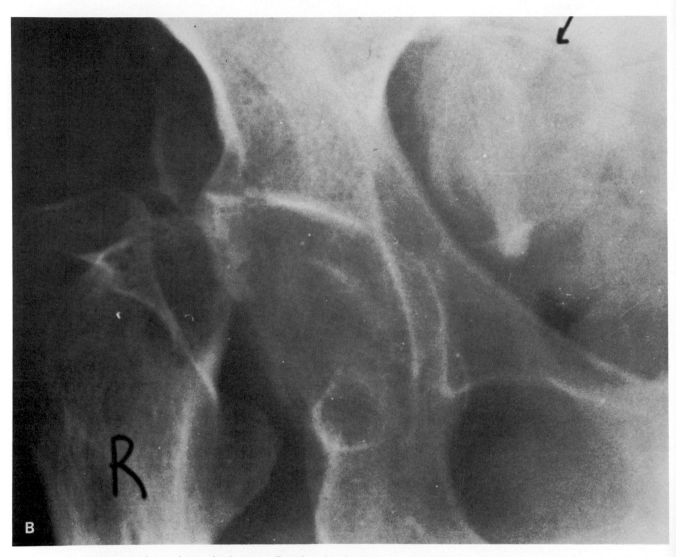

Fig. 4.18 *B,* under general anesthesia the hip was flexed and reduction attempted. Roentgenograms revealed fracture through the neck of the femur. The femoral head was displaced into the pelvis.

COMPLICATIONS

Although no cases of venous obstruction by anterior dislocation were encountered, this complication recently reported by Hampson[44] should be considered if there is a rapid swelling and plethora of the limb. His two cases occurred in pubic dislocations with the femoral head angulating the femoral vein as it pushes against the pelvic rim. Obstruction of the femoral artery has also been reported by the Pennsylvania Orthopaedic Society[82] and Henderson,[49] but none in this series. Early reduction of anterior dislocations should lessen the risk of vascular complications. Supporting the thigh on pillows may partially relieve pressure on the femoral head as mentioned by Hampson.

Although two of the dislocations of the hip with ipsilateral fractures of the femur were recognized at the time of injury, one other dislocation with a severe head injury went unrecognized for 3½ weeks. Since multiple trauma engenders a life-threatening situation which diverts attention from the hip, I have advocated routine roentgenograms of the pelvis in all serious injuries.

In the pubic dislocation in which the neck of the femur was fractured during an attempt at closed reduction, this complication may have been avoided if the hip had been pulled down so that the femoral head was opposite the acetabulum before flexion of the hip was performed.

Avascular necrosis of the femoral head has been reported, although infrequently. This severe complication occurred in only two cases, one having a severe crushing injury and the other avulsing the greater trochanter. It is conceivable that both the medial circumflex iliac and the lateral circumflex iliac arteries were injured with the dislocation.

REDUCTION

Reduction is best performed under a general anesthetic. In the obturator (inferior) type, reduction should be in line with the femur. Gentle flexion of the hip joint with continuous traction and gentle internal rotation and adduction should reduce the hip (Fig. 4.19A–C). In the pubic (superior) type, traction should be in line with the femur, then and only after strong traction sufficient to pull the femoral head distal to the acetabulum, gentle flexion and internal rotation should be applied. No adduction should be attempted until the hip is reduced.

TREATMENT

Just as in posterior dislocations, anterior dislocations require early recognition and prompt reduction under a general anesthetic. Multiple attempts at closed reduction should not be encouraged. If a competent orthopaedist cannot reduce a dislocated hip under a general anesthetic at the first attempt, an open procedure should be performed. Likewise, fragments in the hip joint require an early arthrotomy. Therefore, immediate roentgenograms should be taken after closed reduction. Many of the compressions over the superior-anterior portion of the femoral head are revealed only by the lateral view.

As stated in Chapter 5, Children's Dislocations, and in Chapter 2, Posterior Type I Dislocations, there was no evidence that early weight-bearing increased the percentage of avascular necrosis or traumatic arthritis. The majority of

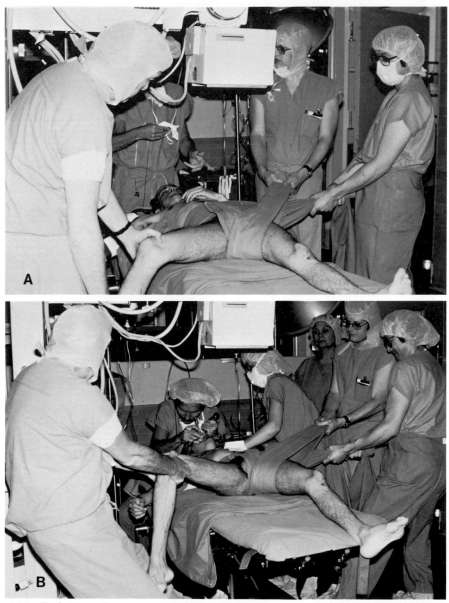

Fig. 4.19 Reduction of an anterior dislocation of the hip (right). Note the wide abduction and external rotation. *A,* reduction under general anesthesia with countertraction. *B,* pull in line of deformity.

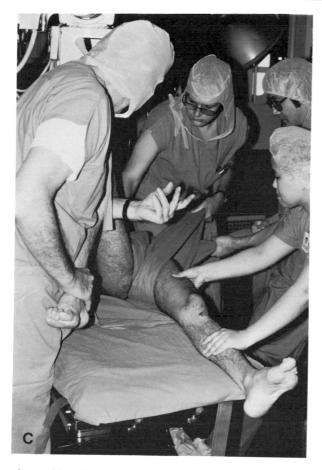

Fig. 4.19 *C,* when femoral head is opposite acetabulum continue traction with hip in flexion.

patients with excellent or good results in the simple obturator dislocations walked by the 2nd month.

Treatment after reduction of the dislocation is immobilization, preferably with balanced skeletal traction. In dislocations with fractures, longer periods of traction may be necessary than the usual 4 to 6 weeks of traction for the simple obturator types.

PROGNOSIS

The majority of simple obturator dislocations without compression fracture of the femoral head have a good prognosis if recognized and reduced promptly on the first attempt, within 24 hours after injury.

A guarded prognosis should be given to those patients having either obturator dislocations with compression fractures of the femoral head or pubic dislocations involving the femoral head, acetabulum, or pubic bones.

Since the results in the anterior dislocations with compression of the femoral head have been unsatisfactory, with resultant traumatic arthritis, it seems justifiable to do an arthrotomy of the hip joint (anterior approach) in all such cases. The reasoning is that small loose fragments of bone and cartilage are displaced into the joint space, leading to an incongruity and eventual traumatic arthritis.

CHAPTER
5

DISLOCATIONS IN CHILDREN

Seventy-five traumatic anterior and posterior dislocations of the hip were seen in 74 patients during a span of 48 years (Tables 1.1–1.3). Included in this group was a bilateral posterior dislocation in a girl 15 years old who died 1 day after injury because of a fat embolism (Fig. 5.1*A*, *B*).

The ages ranged from 2 to 15 years. The age limit of 15 years was chosen since in this group the femoral capital epiphysis was still open.

The children's dislocations represented 9% of the total 830 dislocations in the entire series. Approximately 75% were males and 25% were females, and the right

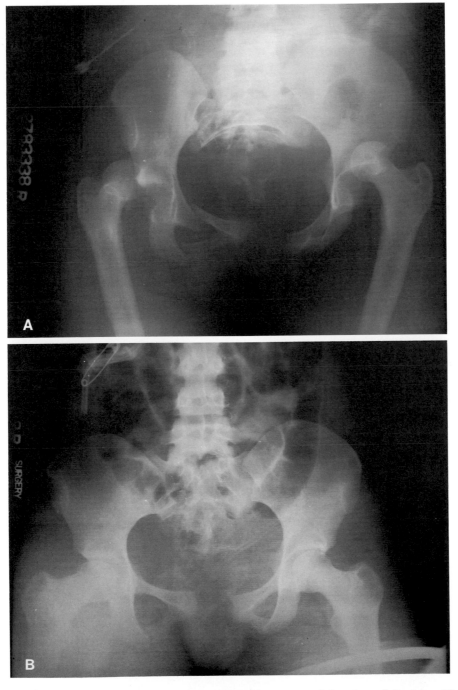

Fig. 5.1 *A*, a 15-year-old girl sustained a bilateral posterior dislocation of the hip with a fracture of the pelvis when she was struck by an automobile. Roentgenogram made the day of injury before reduction. *B*, the hips were reduced under general anesthesia the day of injury by the Allis maneuver, the left reducing easily, the right side requiring two manipulsations before reduction was accomplished. The patient died the next day as a result of fat embolism.

and left hips were about equally involved. There were 11 dislocations in the 2- to 4-year age group, thirteen in the 5- to 7-year group, 18 between 8 and 12 years old, and 33 in the 13- to 15-year-old group. Eight dislocations were anterior and 67 were posterior (59, simple type I); eight were fracture-dislocations. Four of the dislocations had concurrent ipsilateral femoral fractures, three being recognized at the time of injury and one in a 14-year-old was not recognized for 2 ½ months.

The minimum follow-up period and the clinical and roentgenographic criteria are the same as used for the adult dislocations.

CLASSIFICATION OF DISLOCATIONS

The dislocations were divided into anterior and posterior groups, similar to the classification of the adults (see Chapters 2 and 4, on classification). The posterior dislocations were divided into five types (Figs 5.2–5.6). The attitude of a posterior dislocation is shown in Figure 5.7.

The anterior dislocations were all obturator (Figs. 4.2 and 5.8) including one with an ipsilateral femoral fracture recognized at the time of injury (Fig. 4.14A, B).

MECHANISM OF INJURY

The majority of dislocations, both anterior and posterior, occurred following severe trauma. Approximately 60% were due to automobile, motorcycle or bicycle accidents, or occurred when pedestrians were struck by an automobile. As reported by many authors, traumatic dislocations in children tend to occur easily, with minimal trauma, especially in the younger age group. In this series, approximately 30% were due either to falling out of bed, falling down stairs, being pushed by another child, or just tripping. Five dislocations (all posterior) occurred in football games (American) (see Fig. 5.23A, B).

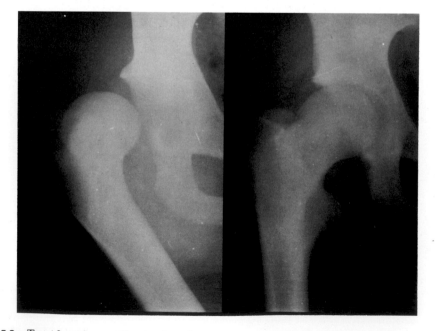

Fig. 5.2   Type I: with or without minor fracture.

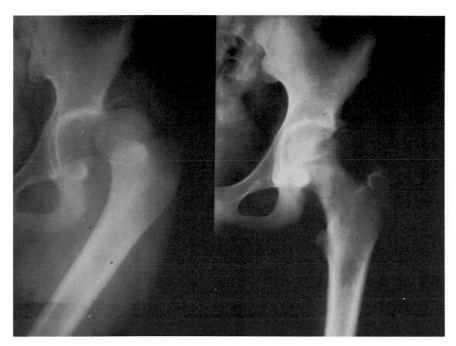

Fig. 5.3 Type II: with a large single fracture of the posterior acetabular rim.

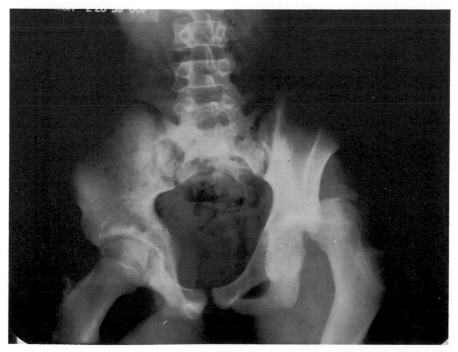

Fig. 5.4 Type III: with a comminuted fracture of the rim of the acetabulum, with or without a major fragment.

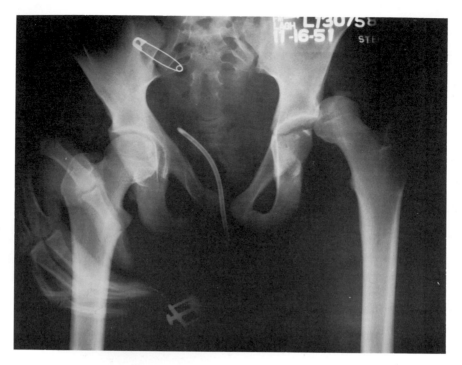

Fig. 5.5   Type IV: with fracture of the acetabular rim and floor.

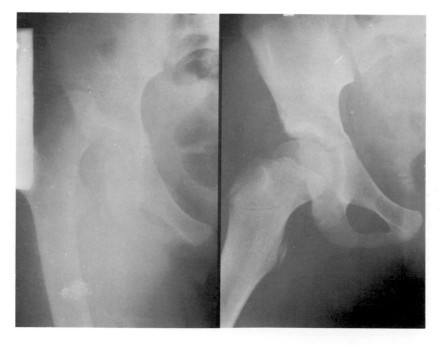

Fig 5.6   Type V: with fracture of the femoral head.

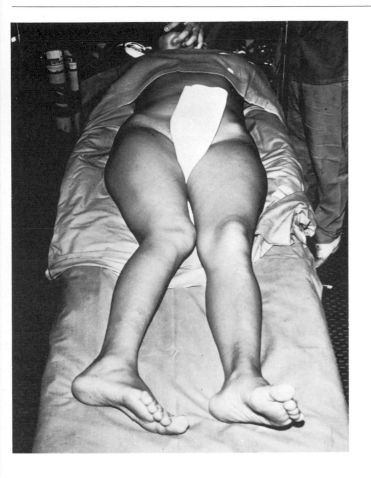

Fig. 5.7   Posterior dislocation, right hip. Note adduction, internal rotation and shortening.

Fig. 5.8   Anterior obturator dislocation, left hip, in a child. Note marked abduction flexion and external rotation of the hip. (From Epstein, H. C.: Traumatic anterior and simple posterior dislocations of the hip in adults and children. In *The American Academy of Orthopaedic Surgeons: Instructional Course Lectures,* vol. 22. The C. V. Mosby Co., St. Louis, 1973. Reproduced with permission.)

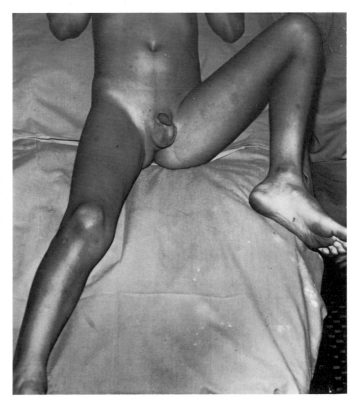

RESULTS

There was sufficient follow-up in 51 dislocations (12 months to 19 ½ years, with an average follow-up of 78.6 months) (Table 5.1).

Open procedures were performed on four patients. One type I in a 3 ½-year-old was opened 7 days after a closed reduction. One type III dislocation in a 14-year-old boy had a primary open procedure with a good result, and another type III injury in a 14-year-old boy was classified as a fair result following an open reduction 2 days after a closed reduction because of instability of the hip. The last patient, previously described, was a 14-year-old girl whose hip was unsuccessfully opened 10 months after a missed diagnosis of a type IV dislocation with an ipsilateral fracture of the femur.

In the anterior dislocations, the results were excellent in six cases (including one with an ipsilateral fracture of the femur) (Fig. 4.14A, B) and good in one. There were no poor or fair results. No compression fractures of the head or acetabular fractures were encountered. All cases were reduced within 24 hours after injury on the first attempt. Five of the patients were fully weight-bearing by the 5th week. The other two patients started late weight-bearing because of fractures of the tibia and femur, respectively. Although avascular necrosis[6] has been reported with anterior dislocations in children none were seen in our series. There were no nerve injuries.

POSTERIOR DISLOCATIONS

The results were as follows: Twenty-four type I dislocations had excellent and 10 had good results (Figs. 5.9A–C; 5.10A–C). Two of the excellent or good results (Table 5.2) were reduced between 25 and 48 hours after injury (Fig. 5.11A, B). The rest were reduced within less than 24 hours after injury. Two of the satisfactory dislocations (Table 5.3) had two attempts at closed reduction (Fig. 5.12A, B); the remaining were reduced on the first attempt.

The four type I dislocations with the fair results were as follows: A 3½-year-old boy (Fig. 5.13A–H) fell in a hole while playing and dislocated his left hip. After reduction under general anesthesia on the day of injury, the joint space on the involved side appeared to be wider than the uninvolved hip. An arthrogram revealed the dislocated side was definitely wider. An open reduction was per-

Table 5.1

Results in 51 Dislocations of the Hip in Children (Ages, 2–15 Years)[a]

Type	Excellent	Good	Fair	Poor	Total
Anterior	6	1	0	0	7
Posterior					
Type I[b]	24	10	4	0	38
Type II	0	0	0	0	0
Type III	0	1	1	1	3
Type IV	0	0	0	2	2
Type V	0	0	1	0	1
Total	30	12	6	3	51
Percentage of results	59%	23%	12%	6%	
		82%			

[a] Average follow-up, 78.6 months.
[b] Type I excellent-good results, 89%.

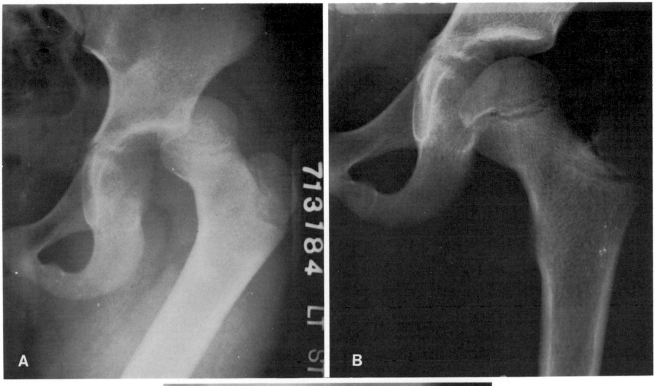

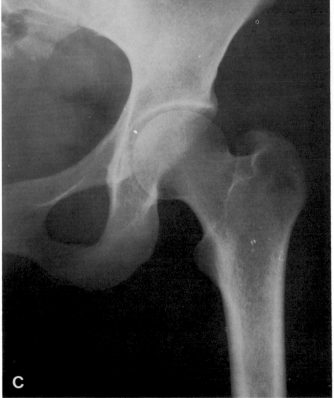

Fig. 5.9 *A*, a 6-year-old male sustained a posterior type I dislocation in an automobile accident. The result was rated excellent 12 years and 4 months later. *B*, a closed reduction was performed on the day of injury. The patient was at bed rest for only 8 days and walked in 2 weeks. *C*, follow-up films 12 years and 4 months later were normal, and patient had normal hip motion. (From Epstein, H. C.: Traumatic anterior and simple posterior dislocations of the hip in adults and children. In *The American Academy of Orthopaedic Surgeons: Instructional Course Lectures*, vol. 22. The C. V. Mosby Co., St. Louis, 1973. Reproduced with permission.)

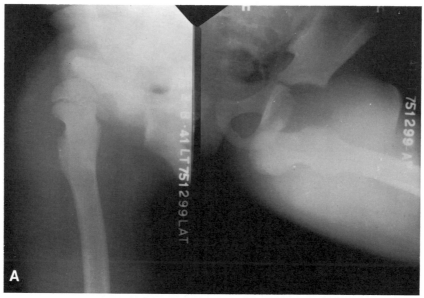

Fig. 5.10 *A*, a 6-year-old boy sustained an anterior dislocation without fracture, with an excellent result. The patient slipped and fell. The dislocation was reduced on the same day and a spica cast was applied. The patient walked in 3 weeks.

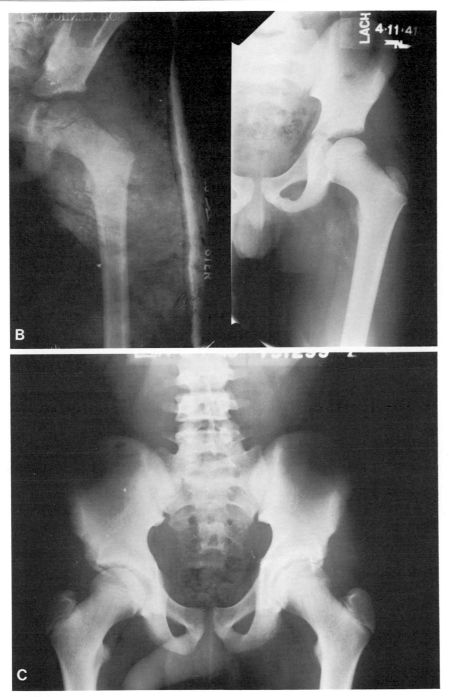

Fig. 5.10 *B,* roentgenogram made two months later. *C,* follow-up roentgenogram made 8½ years later. There was a normal range of hip motion and the patient had no complaints.

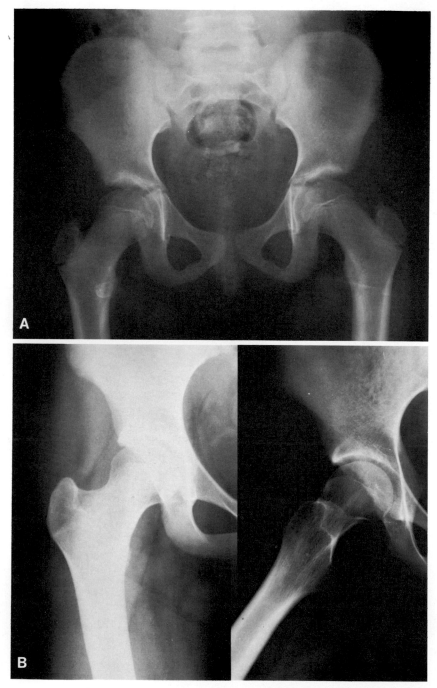

Fig. 5.11   *A*, a 6-year old girl in an automobile vs. automobile accident sustained a type I dislocation of the right hip. The patient had a subdural hematoma and was unconscious. The result after 9½ years was good. *B*, the hip was reduced under general anesthesia at the first attempt by Allis maneuver 48 hours after injury. She was kept in Russell traction 8 weeks and started walking at 2 months. At the last follow-up, age 16 years, the result was good with minimal restriction of motions of the hip and normal x-ray findings.

Table 5.2
Closed Reductions (51 Cases): Number of Hours before Reduction Compared to Outcome

Type	0–24 hr		25–48 hr		49 hr or more		Not reduced[a]		Total
	Excellent or good	Poor or fair	Excellent or good	Poor or fair	Excellent or good	Poor or fair	Excellent or good	Poor or fair	
Anterior	7	0	0	0	0	0	0	0	7
Posterior									
Type I	32	3	2	0	0	0	0	1	38
Type II	0	0	0	0	0	0	0	0	0
Type III	0	2	0	0	0	0	1	0	3
Type IV	0	1	0	0	0	0	0	1	2
Type V	0	0	0	0	0	1	0	0	1
Total	39	6	2	0	0	1	1	2	51

[a] One not reduced (unrecognized); one primary open reduction; one closed and not reduced (opened 7 days later).

Table 5.3
Closed Reductions (47 Dislocations): Number of Reductions Compared to Outcome[a]

Type	One reduction		Two or more reductions		Total	
	Excellent or good	Fair or poor	Excellent or good	Fair or poor	Excellent or good	Fair or poor
Anterior	7	0	0	0	7	0
Type I	32	3	2	0	34	3
Type II	0	0	0	0	0	0
Type III	0	1	0	0	0	1
Type IV	0	1	0	0	0	1
Type V	0	1	0	0	0	1
Total	39	6	2	0	41	6

[a] One never reduced—not recognized (type IV); arthrotomy 10 months after injury; one primary open reduction (type III); one closed followed by open surgery 2 days later (type III); one closed followed by open surgery 7 days later (type I).

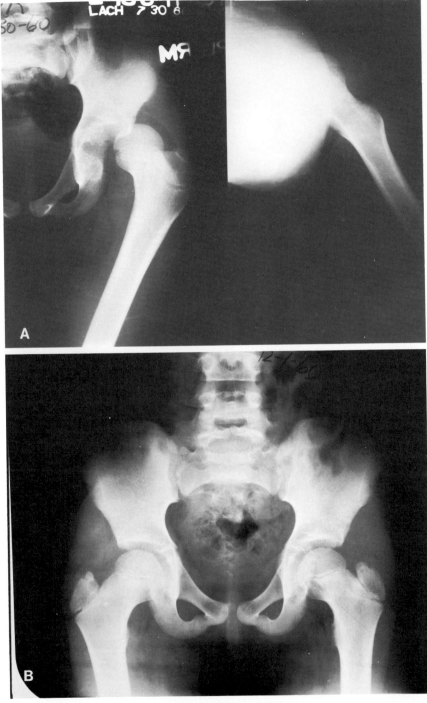

Fig. 5.12　This 8-year-old girl fell while playing and dislocated her left hip. *Two attempts* were made before hip was reduced less than 24 hours after injury under a general anesthetic by the Allis method. Traction was maintained for 3 weeks and the patient was weight-bearing by the 4th week. *A*, This is the roentgenogram before reduction. *B*, the follow-up roentgenogram taken at 13 months. The result was excellent. The patient had a normal pregnancy at the age of 17. (From Epstein, H. C.: Traumatic anterior and simple posterior dislocations of the hip in adults and children. In *The American Academy of Orthopaedic Surgeons: Instructional Course Lectures,* vol. 22. The C. V. Mosby Co., St. Louis, 1973. Reproduced with permission.)

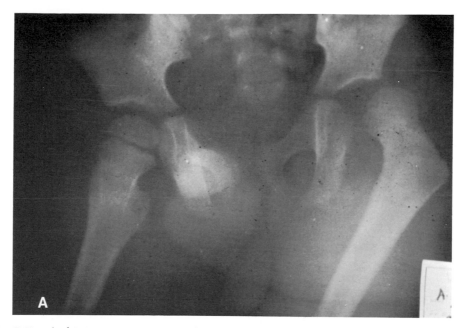

Fig. 5.13 *A*, this is a posterior type I dislocation sustained in this 3½-year-old boy when he fell in a hole. Note the marked internal rotation and adduction of the left hip.

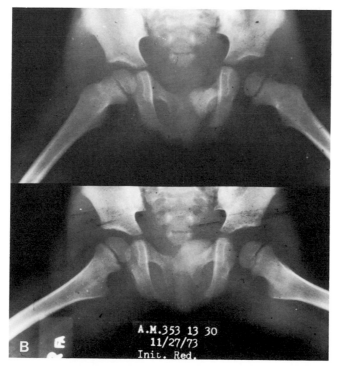

Fig. 5.13 *B*, check films were taken after reduction under a general anesthetic showing a widening of the hip joint space on the involved hip.

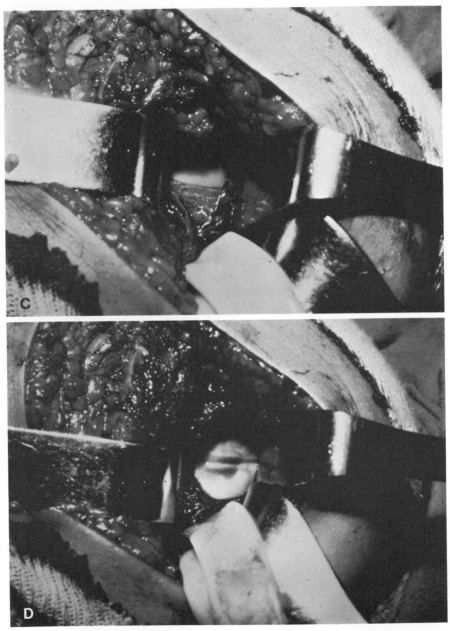

Fig. 5.13 *C* and *D*, at surgery, the femoral head was found to have buttonholed through the capsule. This had to be incised before the hip could be reduced. There was a 2 mm depression over the articular cartilage and a 1 × 1 cm area of slight brownish discoloration of the posterior medial portion of the cartilage of the femoral head. The ligamentum teres was intact, but had a small area of ecchymosis at the insertion into the femoral head.

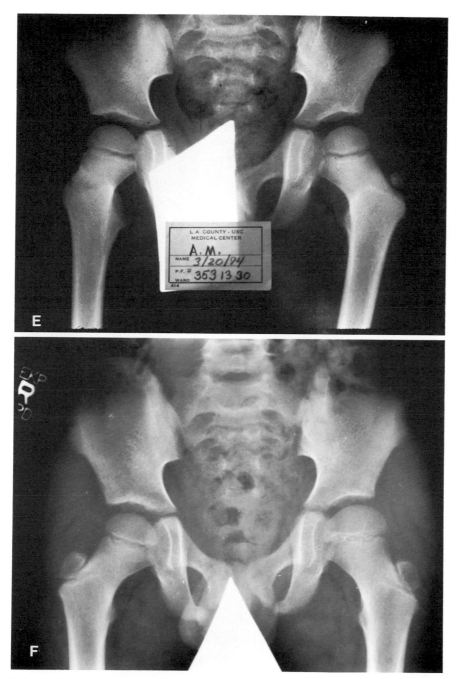

Fig. 5.13 *E*, these are roentgenograms 4 months after injury. Traction was maintained for 3 weeks and the patient was fully ambulatory by the 4th week. Motion of the hip is normal without any complaints. The roentgenograms appear normal. *F*, two years after injury there is a coxa magna of the left hip. Patient walks without a limp and without complaints. There is minimal restriction of motion of the hip.

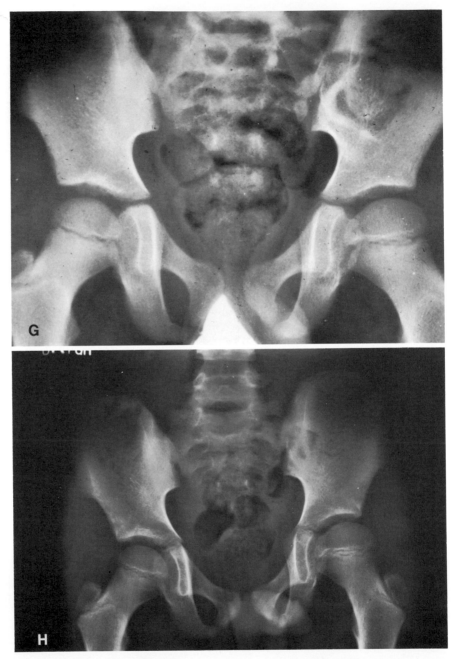

Fig. 5.13 *G*, at 35 months after injury coxa magna is still evident. There are no areas of increased or decreased densities of the femoral head and no segmental collapse. The patient states he has constant hip pain, but walks and runs without a limp. The Trendelenburg is negative. There is approximately 10° of limitation in flexion, abduction, and internal and external rotation of the hip. *H*, at 60 months after injury, coxa magna is more evident. There is valgus deformity of the hip with an approximately ½-inch increase in leg length in the left. Child tires easily after activities. There is a negative Trendelenburg. The left femoral head projects laterally ½ inch out of the acetabulum. There is no segmental collapse of the femoral head.

formed 7 days after injury and revealed that the femoral head had buttonholed through the capsule. The posterior band of the capsule had to be incised before the hip could be reduced. The articular cartilage of the head had a 2-mm depression and a 1 × 1 cm area of brownish discoloration of the posterior medial portion of the cartilage. The ligamentum teres was not ruptured although a small area of ecchymosis was noted at the insertion into the acetabular wall. After surgery, the child was placed in balanced traction for 3 weeks and then started weight-bearing. At follow-up 4 months later, the left femoral head appeared normal. Two years after injury there was definite coxa magna with some widening of the femoral neck. At follow-up 66 months after injury, the left femoral head appeared to be larger than the uninvolved side with the neck definitely wider and shorter. There were no areas of increased or decreased densities of the femoral head and no segmental collapse. The epiphysial line revealed irregularity and widening. At the last examination, 5 years after injury, there was more enlargement of the left femoral head, and the involved lower extremity was ½ inch longer as measured from the anterior iliac spine to the medial malleolus. The hip was in a coxa valgus position as well as coxa magna. There was no irregularity or depression of the femoral head and no areas of increased or decreased densities. The examination revealed a slight limp on the left side after walking 50 feet. The mother stated the child tired easily after playing at school. The Trendelenburg was negative, there was a ¼-inch atrophy of the involved extremity, and motion of the left hip was restricted minimally.

In discussing dislocations of the hip in children presented by Funk,[31] Gartland, in a report of the Pennsylvania Society,[82] stated that he recently heard about two fresh dislocations in children under 5 years of age in whom closed reduction proved impossible. At open reduction, in both cases, the femoral head was found to have buttonholed through the capsule. The final result in these two cases was not stated. Glass and Powell,[36] reporting on complications of traumatic dislocations in children, described six cases with development of an enlarged femoral head. In two of the dislocations, open procedures were performed. Three children were under the age of 5 years; the other two were 11 and 13 years, respectively. They stated that this complication may lead to osteoarthritis in later life.

The second case is that of a 15-year-old young man involved in an automobile accident, incurring a dislocation of his left hip (Fig. 5.14A, B). It was reduced the day of injury by the Allis method under im morphine sulfate. H & P suspension was maintained for 6 weeks and then full weight-bearing. There was minimal weakness of the extensor digitorum longus upon discharge. Six months after injury there was premature closure of the upper femoral epiphysis. At the last examination, 2 years postinjury, he was rated as a fair result because of the intermittent pain in his left hip, painful paresthesias over the dorsum of the foot and, weakness of the extensor digitorum longus. Roentgenograms revealed minimal osteophytes superiorly and inferiorly at the junction of the head and neck and minimal narrowing of the joint space.

The third patient is a 15-year-old girl who sustained a dashboard dislocation of her left hip (Fig. 5.15A, B), with a laceration and undisplaced fracture of the ipsilateral patella. Reduction of the dislocation was accomplished easily under a general anesthetic by the Allis maneuver and the patient was placed in balanced traction for 1 month, followed by full weight-bearing. At follow-up, 6 months after injury, she was asymptomatic, except when sitting for a prolonged period of time. This pain was relieved by walking. Roentgenograms at that time appeared to be normal. Follow-up at 3 years revealed occasional aching in the left hip lasting for a few hours to a day. She was able to sit through two theater features without

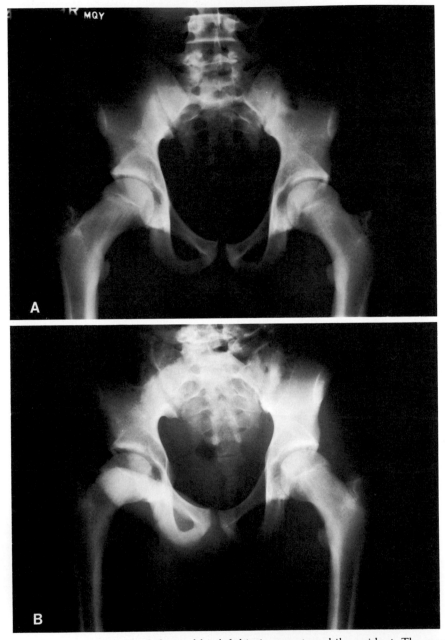

Fig. 5.14 A 15-year-old male dislocated his left hip in an automobile accident. The result 2 years after injury is fair. *A*, this is a type I dislocation of the left hip reduced closed by the Allis method on the day of injury. Traction was maintained for 6 weeks and then full weight-bearing. There was minimal weakness of the extensor digitorum longus on discharge. *B*, two years postinjury, the patient complains of intermittent left hip pain with painful paresthesias over the dorsum of the foot and weakness of the extensor digitorum longus.

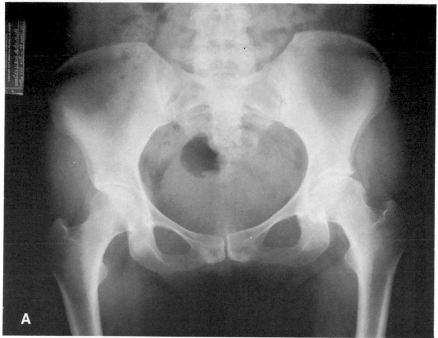

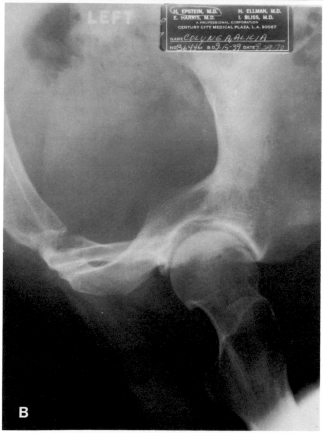

Fig. 5.15 *A*, this 15-year-old girl dislocated her left hip in an automobile accident. The hip was reduced easily on the day of injury by the Allis method. She was kept in traction for 5 weeks, then full weight-bearing. There was a laceration of the knee with an undisplaced patellar fracture. *B*, at follow-up 9 years postinjury, the rating was good. At 16½ years the rating was changed to fair because of traumatic arthritis of the hip with narrowing of the joint space and spur formation at the superior and inferior head and neck junction. There was definite limitation of hip motion. There is a limp on walking and patient has pain and discomfort in the involved hip.

discomfort. She walked without a limp, with a negative Trendelenburg. There was only minimal restriction of motion of the left hip and no atrophy of the thigh. Roentgenograms revealed a normal joint space and there was no evidence of avascular necrosis. There was a small ossicle of bone medially, probably over the fovea. Nine years after injury the patient was reexamined. There were no complaints about her injured hip and motion was only minimally restricted. Roentgenograms were not taken at this time because the patient was pregnant, but those taken after her pregnancy terminated revealed no change over those taken at the 3-year follow-up.

The last follow-up was 16 years and 9 months after injury. The roentgenogram revealed the loose fragment medially, although on the lateral view it appeared to be outside the hip joint. The joint space was normal with definite spur formation on the superior and inferior portions of the head-neck junction. There were also two small areas of decreased density in the center of the femoral head. Clinically, pain started in the left hip when walking, developed suddenly, and lasted approximately 15 minutes. "The hip seems to go out of the socket." Examination revealed a definite limp, left hip, ½-inch atrophy of the thigh, and a range of motion as follows:

	Right	Left
Flexion	130°	110°
Abduction	50°	40°
Internal Rotation	25°	10°
External Rotation	35°	10°
Adduction	20°	20°
Extension	10°	5°

The fourth case is that of a 12-year-old male who sustained a posterior dislocation of his left hip in an auto vs. auto accident (Fig. 5.16A–D). The hip was reduced the day of injury on the first attempt under general anesthesia at another hospital, and he was transferred to LAC-USC Medical Center, where he was placed in balanced traction. One week later the patient complained of pain in the opposite hip and roentgenograms revealed a grade II slipped femoral capital epiphysis. This was pinned with four Hagie pins. At follow-up 6 years later for his slipped femoral capital epiphysis, roentgenograms of the traumatically dislocated hip revealed some flattening of the lateral head of the femur with minimal narrowing of the hip joint. The range of motion was equal to that on the opposite side. The rating of fair was based on the roentgenographic findings.

FRACTURE-DISLOCATIONS

The results in the six fracture-dislocations were as follows: Of three type III injuries, there was one good, one fair, and one poor result.

The one good result was a 14-year-old male who dislocated his left hip when struck by an automobile while riding a bicycle. A primary open reduction was performed the day of injury. Many fragments were removed from the hip joint and a large superior acetabular lip was repositioned with two screws. Some bloody infiltration was noted in the sheath of the sciatic nerve but there was no paralysis. Balanced traction was maintained for 1 month, then full weight-bearing. At follow-up, 4½ years later, there was a normal-appearing hip joint with two screws inserted into the superior acetabular lip. The patient was rated good instead of excellent because there was 10° limitation on external rotation of the hip (Fig. 5.17A, B).

The case with a fair result was that of a 15-year-old boy involved in an automobile accident. The dislocation was reduced closed on the day of injury.

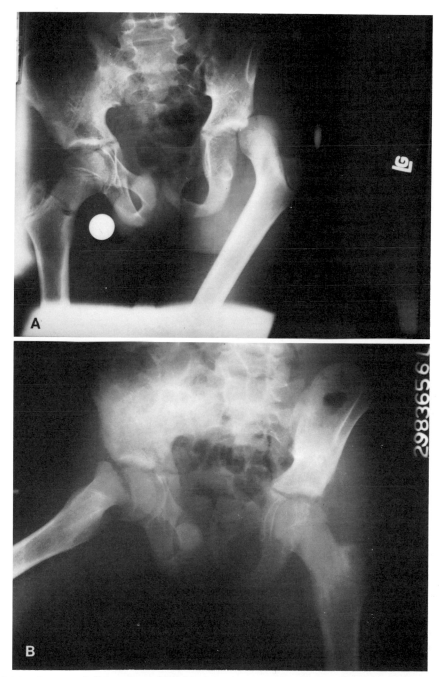

Fig. 5.16   *A*, a type I dislocation of left hip in a 12-year-old male involved in an auto vs. auto accident; right hip appears normal. Dislocation was reduced closed under a general anesthetic the day of injury at another hospital. The result 6 years later was rated fair. *B*, roentgenograms 7 days after reduction of the left hip. The patient complained of pain in the right hip and roentgenograms revealed a grade II slipped femoral capital epiphysis.

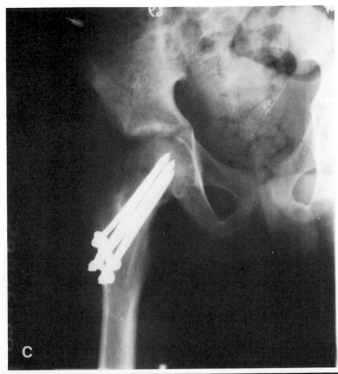

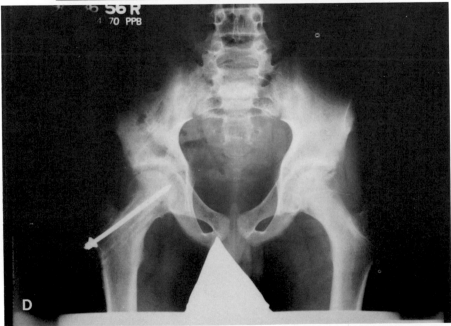

Fig. 5.16 *C*, the right hip was pinned, using four Hagie pins. *D*, six years after his injury the left hip is rated fair because of flattening of the femoral head laterally. Motion of the left hip is equal to that of the right hip.

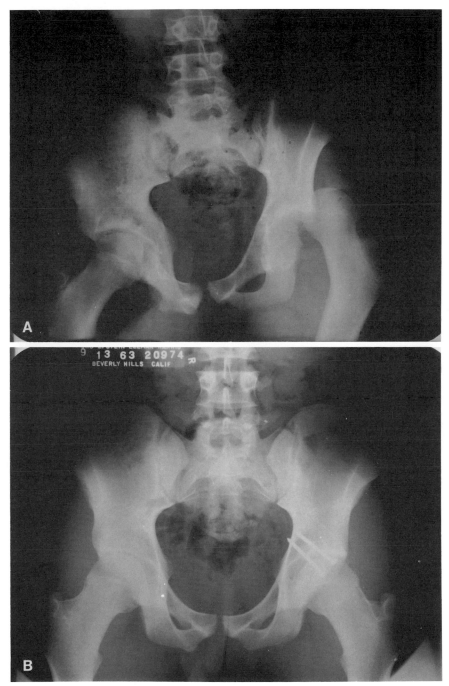

Fig. 5.17 *A*, this 14-year-old boy sustained a type III posterior dislocation of the left hip when struck by an automobile while riding his bicycle. A primary open reduction was performed on the day of injury. The roentgenogram reveals posterior dislocation with multiple fractures of the acetabulum. *B*, these are roentgenograms made 4 years and 7 months after injury. At surgery a posterior approach was made and many free fragments were removed from the hip joint. A 3 × 2 cm piece of posterior superior acetabular rim fragment was anatomically repositioned by two screws. Balanced traction was used for 1 month and weight-bearing started 4 months after injury. Although patient has no pain and walked without a limp he is rated as good rather than excellent because of 10° limitation on external rotation of the hip. (From Epstein, H. C.: Traumatic anterior and simple posterior dislocations of the hip in adults and children. In *The American Academy of Orthopaedic Surgeons: Instructional Course Lectures,* vol. 22. The C. V. Mosby Co., St. Louis, 1973. Reproduced with permission.)

However, the hip was unstable and an open reduction was performed the following day. Fragments were found in the hip joint and a large acetabular fragment was repositioned with two screws; balanced traction was maintained for 6 weeks. Three years later there was spur formation at the junction of the head and neck superiorly and moderately, with limitation of hip motion and discomfort in the hip. There was ½ inch of atrophy of the thigh on the involved side (Fig. 5.18A–C).

The poor result occurred in a 15-year-old boy who was involved in an automobile accident. The hip was reduced the same day at another hospital and the patient was transferred to the LAC-USC Medical Center. After reduction it was noted that the joint space was wider on the reduced hip, but no further surgery was performed. Treatment consisted of 10 days of Russell's traction and 10 days of non-weight-bearing. There had been pain from the beginning of weight-bearing. Roentgenograms at 10 months postinjury revealed early changes of avascular necrosis, and at 16 months there was compression of the weight-bearing portion of the femoral head with areas of increased and decreased densities. The patient was having moderate pain in his hip with moderate limitation of motion and he needed crutches for weight-bearing (Fig. 5.19A–D).

Of the two type IV dislocations, both were classified as having a poor result.

A 14-year-old girl sustained a type IV fracture in an accident with dislocation of the right hip and a fracture of the ipsilateral femur. There was also cerebral concussion and sciatic paralysis. The dislocation of the hip was not recognized until approximately 2½ months later, when roentgenograms were taken of the pelvis to determine the progress of the healing femoral fracture. Ten months after injury an attempt was made to reduce the dislocated hip by arthrotomy but this proved unsuccessful because of severe soft tissue contractions. She was last seen at the hospital at the age of 19, when she delivered a normal child (Fig. 5.20).

The second type IV fracture-dislocation occurred in a 15-year-old girl struck by an automobile. There was a fracture of the opposite pelvis, a perforated bladder, and a tear of the mesentery. A closed reduction was accomplished just prior to abdominal surgery. Russell's traction was maintained for 1 month. She started full weight-bearing at 3 months. At follow-up, approximately 13½ years after injury, there were 1½ inches of atrophy of the thigh on the involved side, with moderate limitation of hip motion and with discomfort in the hip after driving her car for 20 minutes. Roentgenograms revealed avascular necrosis with advanced osteoarthritis. The patient has had five children and does her own housework but has to rest frequently (Fig. 5.21A–C).

There was one type V fracture-dislocation with a fair result (Fig. 5.22A, B). This occurred in a 6-year-old girl who was involved in an automobile accident. Reduction was performed the day after injury when the patient stated that the doctor grabbed her hip and pulled it, without any anesthesia. The patient was then put in an abduction frame for 3 months, then full weight-bearing. At follow-up, 13 years and 5 months later, the roentgenograms revealed that the head fragment had reattached to the neck to form an exostotic mass blocking full flexion and adduction motion. No surgical treatment was advised.

All excellent or good results in children's dislocations were in either anterior or posterior type I dislocations, except for a type III that had a primary open procedure (Fig. 5.17A, B). This gives an 82% incidence of excellent-good results. Eliminating type III dislocation, the incidence of excellent-good results is 81%.

The excellent-good results according to the different age groups are as follows:

Age 2–4, two of three cases (67%).

Age 5–7, 11 of 11 cases (100%).

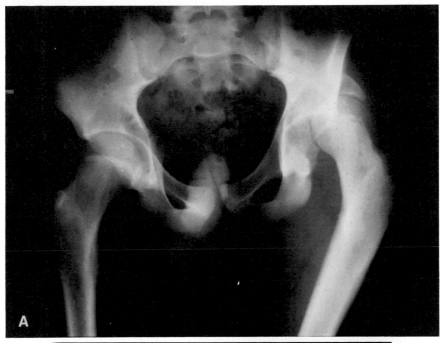

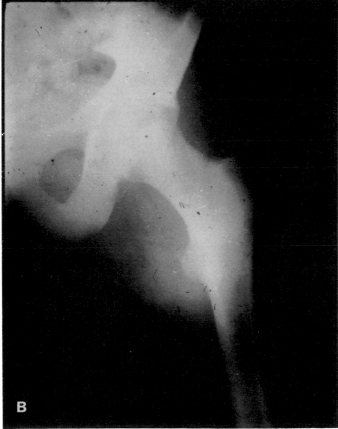

Fig. 5.18 *A*, this 15-year-old boy sustained a posterior type III dislocation of the left hip when involved in an automobile accident. Roentgenograms reveal a posterior dislocation with a comminuted fragment off the superior acetabular rim. *B*, the dislocation was reduced closed under general anesthetic, on the same day; however, it was unstable. An open reduction was performed the following day. Fragments were found within the joint. The large acetabular fragment was repositioned anatomically with two screws. (From Epstein, H. C.: Traumatic anterior and simple posterior dislocations of the hip in adults and children. In *The American Academy of Orthopaedic Surgeons: Instructional Course Lectures,* vol. 22. The C. V. Mosby Co., St. Louis, 1973. Reproduced with permission.)

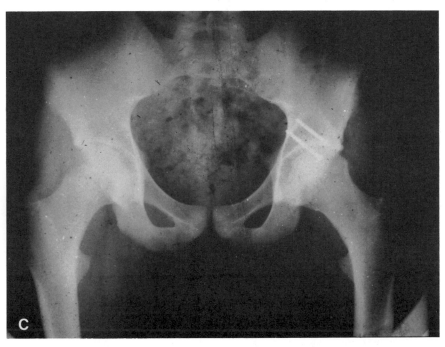

Fig. 5.18 C, roentgenograms made at follow-up 3 years later showed the hip to be reduced; the acetabular fragment contains two screws. There is spur formation at the superior and inferior borders of the head and neck junction. The patient has moderate limitation of hip motion with discomfort. The result is fair. (From Epstein, H. C.: Traumatic anterior and simple posterior dislocations of the hip in adults and children. In *The American Academy of Orthopaedic Surgeons: Instructional Course Lectures,* vol. 22. The C. V. Mosby Co., St. Louis, 1973. Reproduced with permission.)

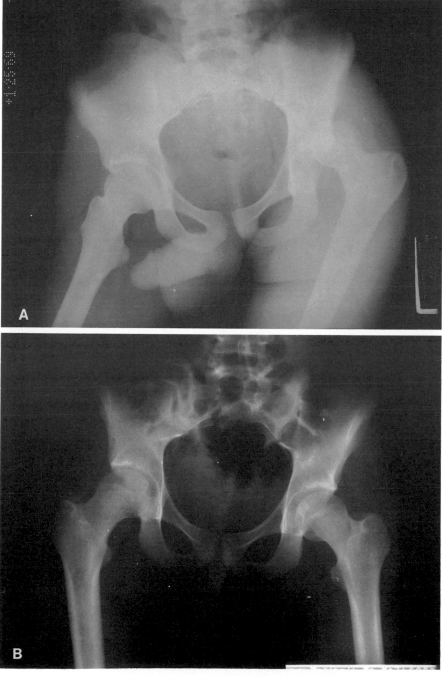

Fig. 5.19 *A*, a 15-year-old male sustained a type III dislocation of the hip in an automobile accident. Thirteen months after injury the result is rated as poor with evidence of avascular necrosis. Roentgenograms show a posterior type III dislocation. Note the fragment about the joint. *B*, the hip was reduced the same day at another hospital and the patient was transferred to LAC/USC Medical Center. Note the widening of the joint space of the left hip compared to the right. He was kept in traction for 3 months and started on weight-bearing at 8 months.

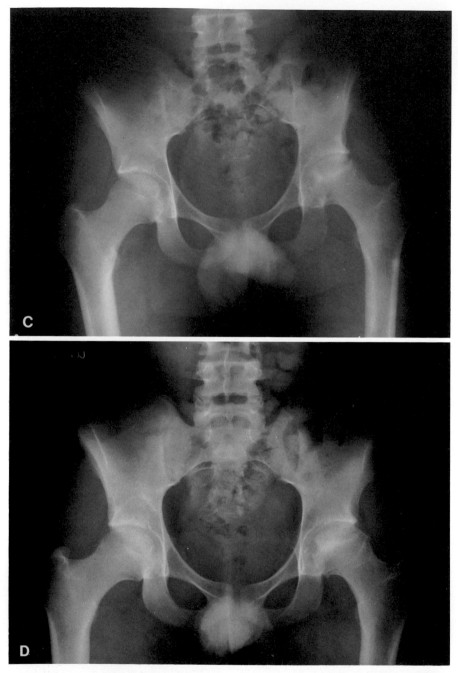

Fig. 5.19 *C*, at 10 months there are early changes of avascular necrosis with compression of the weight-bearing portion of the femoral head with areas of increased and decreased densities. *D*, anteroposterior roentgenograms at 13 months reveal more advanced changes of avascular necrosis, with depression of the devitalized head, sclerosis, and moderate osteophytes at the junction of the head and neck, superiorly and inferiorly. There was moderate limitation of hip motion and moderate hip pain.

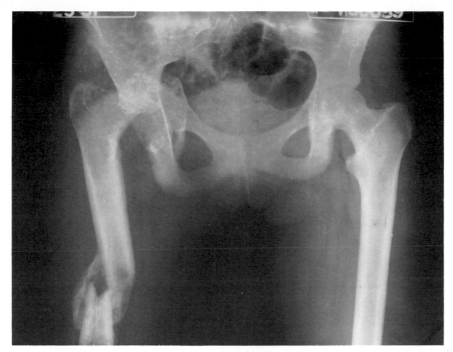

Fig. 5.20 A 14-year-old girl in an automobile accident sustained a type IV fracture-dislocation of the right hip and a fracture of the ipsilateral femur. There was also cerebral concussion with sciatic paralysis. The dislocation of the hip was not recognized until approximately 3 months later when this roentgenogram of the pelvis was made to determine the progress of the healing femoral fracture. Ten months after injury an attempt was made to reduce the dislocated hip by arthrotomy but this proved unsuccessful because of severe soft tissue contractures. The result was rated poor. She was last seen at the hospital at the age of 18, when she delivered a normal child.

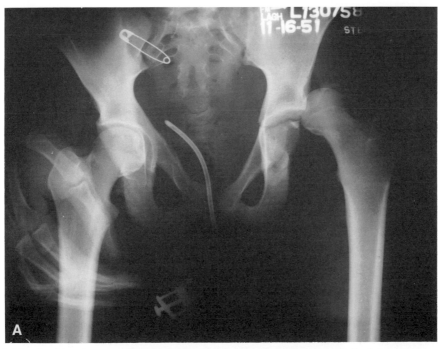

Fig. 5.21 *A*, this 15-year-old girl sustained this type IV dislocation of the left hip when she was struck by an automobile. There was a fracture of the right hemipelvis, a rupture of the bladder, and a tear of the mesentery. (From Epstein, H. C.: Traumatic anterior and simple posterior dislocations of the hip in adults and children. In *The American Academy of Orthopaedic Surgeons: Instructional Course Lectures,* vol. 22. The C. V. Mosby Co., St. Louis, 1973. Reproduced with permission.)

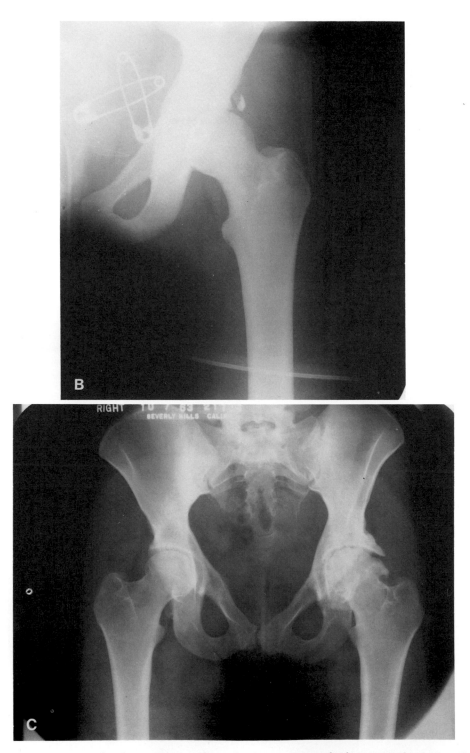

Fig. 5.21 *B*, a closed reduction was performed prior to surgery for her internal injuries. She was maintained in traction for 1 month and started weight-bearing at 3 months. *C*, at 12 years after injury there is avascular necrosis with pain and moderate limitation of the hip motion. Her result is classified as poor. She has five children and does her own housework, but because of discomfort in the hip she needs frequent rest periods.

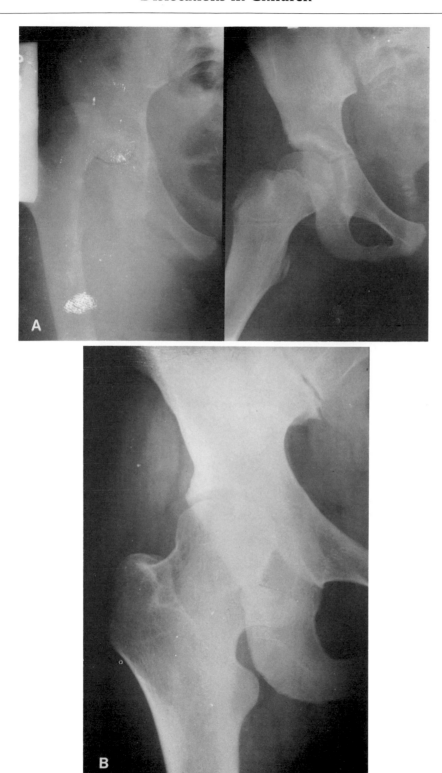

Fig. 5.22 *A*, a 6-year-old girl sustained a type V dislocation with a fracture of the femoral head. The result was rated fair. Patient was injured in an automobile accident. The dislocation was reduced by traction the day after injury. She was in an abduction frame for 3 months and was able to walk after that. *B*, roentgenograms made 13 years and 5 months later. The head fragment had evidently reattached itself to the neck of the femur, forming an exostotic mass blocking full flexion and adduction motion. Because of this the case was rated as fair. No surgical treatment was advised.

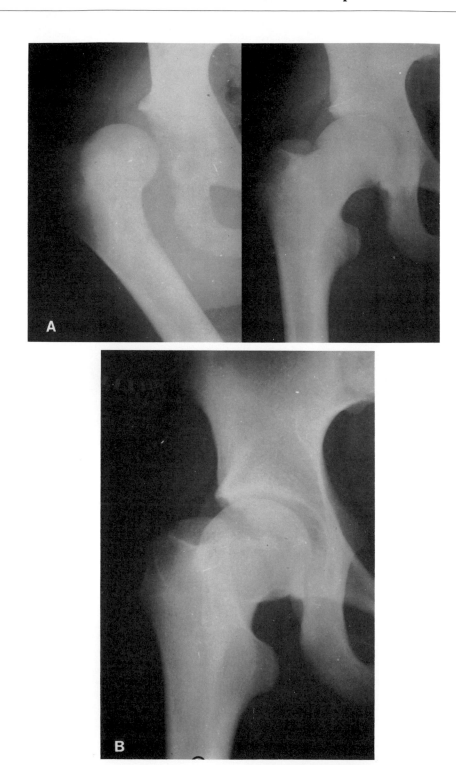

Fig. 5.23 *A*, a 14-year-old male sustained a posterior dislocation of the hip when tackled during a football game. The result is rated excellent 4 years later. Roentgenograms made before and after closed reduction. The hip was reduced under Pentothal anesthesia by the Allis maneuver. Buck's traction was applied for 2 weeks and the patient was up on crutches at 2 months. *B*, roentgenograms made at the last follow-up reveal a normal-appearing hip with all the epiphyses closed. The patient had a normal range of motion without complaints.

Age 8–12, 12 of 12 cases (100%).

Age 13–15, 17 of 25 cases (68%).

However, the statistics can be misleading since an open reduction was performed in a 3½-year-old whose hip had buttonholed through the capsule (Fig. 5.13A–H), and all the fracture-dislocations occurred in older children whose hips sustained a more severe type of trauma.

ROENTGENOGRAPHIC JOINT CHANGES

Nine of the 51 dislocations with sufficient follow-up revealed roentgenographic joint changes (Table 5.4). Avascular necrosis occurred in three dislocations (6%), and traumatic arthritis was evident in six dislocations (12%). There were no cases of myositis ossificans. Although avascular necrosis has been reported in anterior dislocations in children, none was evident in this series and there was no traumatic arthritis.

The one type I avascular necrosis in a child was so called because of a coxa magna following open reduction. Sixty-six months after injury the head was still enlarged. Time will tell whether this femoral head will show all the changes of avascular necrosis. The other dislocations with avascular necrosis occurred in a type III dislocation in which the joint space was widened after reduction, and in a type IV dislocation with multiple injuries.

One of the patients with a type I dislocation with traumatic arthritis was rated good at 9 years and fair at 19½ years. The other two were reduced within 14 hours after injury, on the first attempt, in a 12- and 15-year-old, respectively.

NERVE INJURIES

Three nerve injuries were associated with dislocations, two in a type I injury and one in a type IV injury. All were sciatic. One type I with paralysis still had weakness in the great toe extensor after 21 years. The other two returned to normal by the end of 1 year. The most important factor in the production of nerve injury in type I dislocations may be the marked internal rotation of the hip which occurs at the time of dislocation. This rotation causes a winding and tightening of the sciatic nerve. In the type IV dislocation, the most probable cause of nerve injury could be direct pressure on the sciatic nerve caused by the femoral head or an acetabular fragment (see Chapter 11, Nerve Injuries).

Nerve injuries in dislocations of the hip in children are rare. Pearson and Mann[80] reported on five such cases, all in posterior dislocations, with only one returning to normal. The remaining four had some degree of weakness or paresthesias of the foot. In one case an open reduction was performed 3 months

Table 5.4
Roentgenographic Joint Changes in Nine Fair or Poor Results in Children

Type	Avascular necrosis	Traumatic arthritis
Type I	1[a]	3
Type II	0	0
Type III	1	1
Type IV	1	1
Type V	0	1
Total	3	6
Percentage	6%	12%

[a] Coxa magna; hip buttonholed through capsule; opened 7 days after injury.

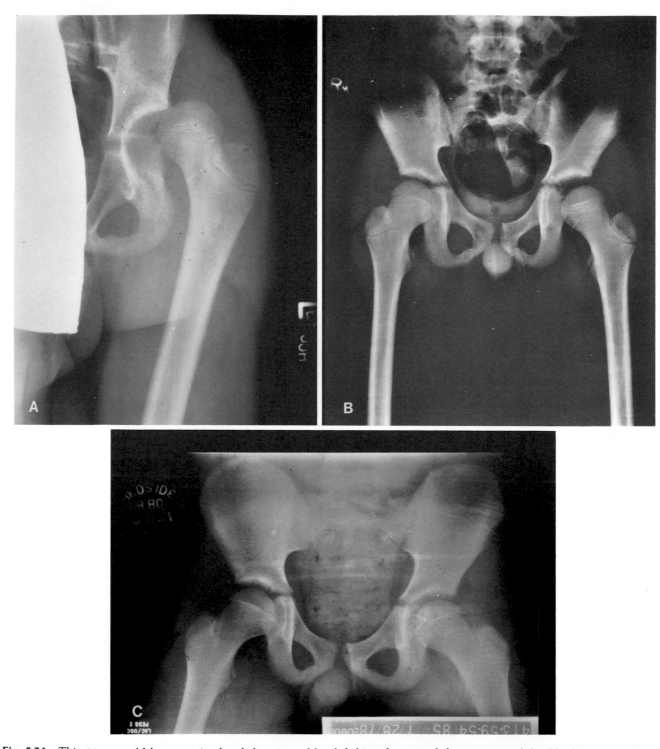

Fig. 5.24 This 11-year-old boy sustained a dislocation of his left hip when struck by an automobile. The hip was reduced closed on the day of injury under general anesthetic. Check roentgenograms after reduction revealed a wide joint space on the involved side. An open reduction done immediately revealed the acetabular labrum to have been invaginated into the acetabulum; this was teased out and replaced anatomically. Five months after injury there are early signs of avascular necrosis. The result is fair (this case is not included in the final statistics). *A*, posterior type I dislocation. *B*, after reduction the left hip reveals a wider joint space. *C*, after open reduction roentgenogram taken shows a normal joint space.

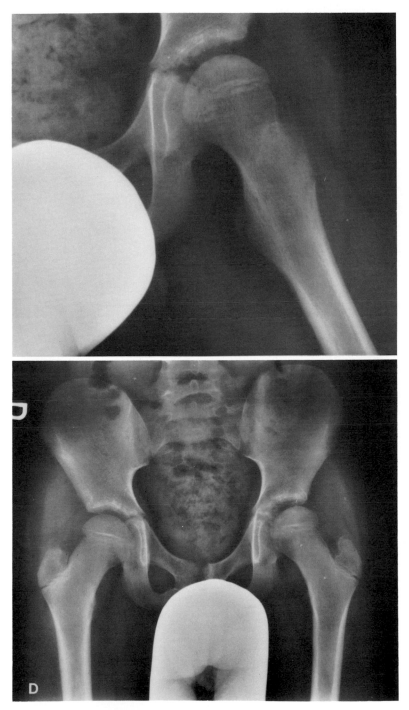

Fig. 5.24 *D*, anterior-posterior and lateral roentgenograms taken 5 months after injury. There is lateral displacement of the femoral head with areas of increased density. The patient has slight pain and limps with weight-bearing. There is ½ inch of atrophy of the left thigh with minimal limitation of hip motion.

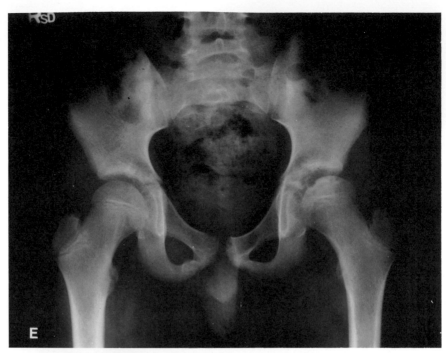

Fig. 5.24 *E,* anterior-posterior and lateral roentgenograms taken 10 months after injury reveals more definite evidence of avascular necrosis. There is irregularity of the femoral head with areas of increased and decreased densities. There is suggestion of a segmental collapse of the weight-bearing portion of the femur with more lateral displacement out of the acetabulum. The patient complains of intermittent hip pain. There is 1 inch of atrophy of the left thigh; internal and external rotation of the hip is, now, restricted approximately 50% of normal, and flexion and abduction are restricted 25% of normal.

Table 5.5
Anterior and Posterior Type I Dislocations of Hip (45 Cases): Period Before Full Weight-Bearing Compared to Outcome

Time in weeks	Anterior		Posterior		Total	
	Exceellent or good	Fair or poor	Excellent or good	Fair or poor	Excellent or good	Fair or poor
3–4	2	0	15	0	17	0
5–6	3	0	10	2	13	2
7–8	0	0	4	2	4	2
8–10	1	0	4	0	5	0
More than 12	1	0	1	0	2	0
Total	7	0	34	4	41	4

after dislocation, but no statement was made as to what was found. Schlonsky and Miller[91] reported two cases of sciatic paralysis, one with an ipsilateral fracture of the femur. Both returned to normal at 38 months.

Gartland reported one case of sciatic palsy in the final report of the Pennsylvania Orthopaedic Society.[82] This did not influence the end result, so apparently the paralysis returned to normal.

It was an interesting observation that approximately 30% of these dislocations were caused by what one would call trivial injuries, such as falling down, being pushed, or just tripping. No displasias of the acetabulum were encountered and there were no recurrent dislocations. In contrast to congenital dislocations, of which the majority occur in girls, traumatic dislocations occurred in 75% of males. So-called trivial injuries do not necessarily mean that the reduction can be accomplished easily. The one type I posterior dislocation which proved difficult to reduce closed occurred in a 3½-year-old child who fell into a hole.

This study indicates that early weight-bearing (Table 5.5) did not increase the complication of avascular necrosis or traumatic arthritis. The majority of the patients with anterior and simple posterior dislocations walked by the 6th week. At least one-third of those with excellent results were walking by the 3rd week (Figs. 5.25 and 5.26A, B).

Just as with adults, it is important to reduce a dislocation at the first attempt. Simple anterior and posterior dislocations reduced gently on the initial attempt 24 hours after injury invariably had excellent or good results.

Fracture-dislocations of the hip in children require the same type of treatment advocated for adults.

In our small series of fracture-dislocations, our only good result was obtained after primary open reduction of the hip joint and removal of fragments in a type III dislocation.

Not included in the statistics because of insufficient follow-up are two fracture-dislocations in which loose fragments were removed from the hip joint in a 12-year-old male and a 13-year-old male, respectively.

Roentgenograms of the pelvis should be taken after reduction of a dislocation in order to determine whether there is a concentric reduction. If the hip on the involved side reveals a widened joint space one should consider an immediate arthrotomy. In two such cases, one type I (Fig. 5.27A–C) and a type III dislocation (Fig. 5.19A–D), check roentgenograms revealed a wider joint space after reduction, but no arthrotomy was performed.

Canale and Manugian[12a] reported recently on irreducible traumatic dislocations of the hip. They described buttonholing of the femoral head through the capsule and a displaced piriformis muscle preventing a closed reduction. In one of our cases an inverted limbus was a cause of an irreducible hip (Fig. 5.24A–E), and an osteocartilaginous loose fragment was the cause of a nonconcentric reduction. In both dislocations an arthrotomy was performed with a poor result in one and a fair result in the other.

Glass and Powell[36] described 14 complications in their series of 47 dislocations in children. Six of these were enlarged femoral heads. Although no etiology was discussed, these authors believed that this condition may lead to osteoarthritis in later life.

Ferguson and Howarth[29a] thought coxa magna to be due to a compensatory increase in blood supply to the hip joint as a result of a reactive hyperemia following an initial ischemic catastrophy. Brighton[8] believes the circulation to the femoral head is compromised during the period of time that the hip was dislocated and that a mild degree of ischemia might lead to increased bone growth in the femoral head because of a contemporary increase in blood supply. Siffert[93]

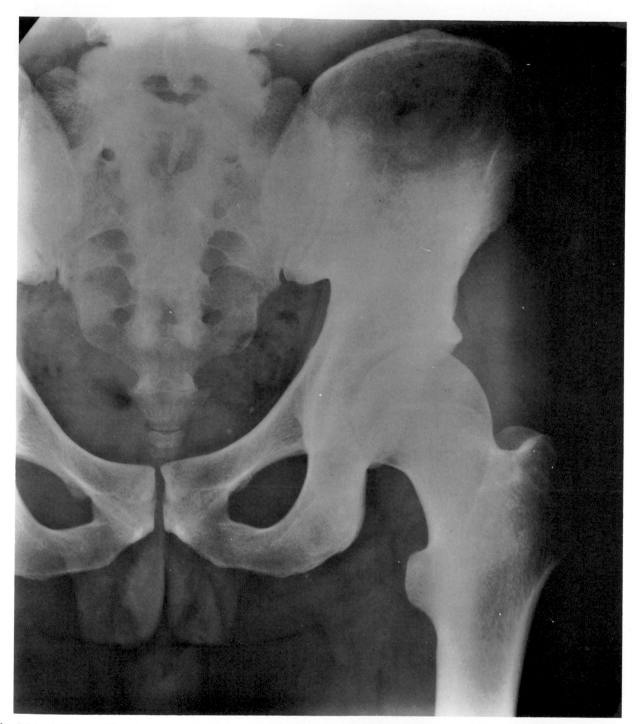

Fig. 5.25 A 7-year-old male sustained a dislocated right hip when an automobile ran over him. The result was excellent 18 years and 3 months later. The hip was reduced the day of injury at another hospital under general anesthesia. His legs were tied together for 8 days and he walked in 2 weeks. At follow-up examination the patient has no complaints. Range of motion is normal and roentgenograms are normal. The patient has been a professional boxer.

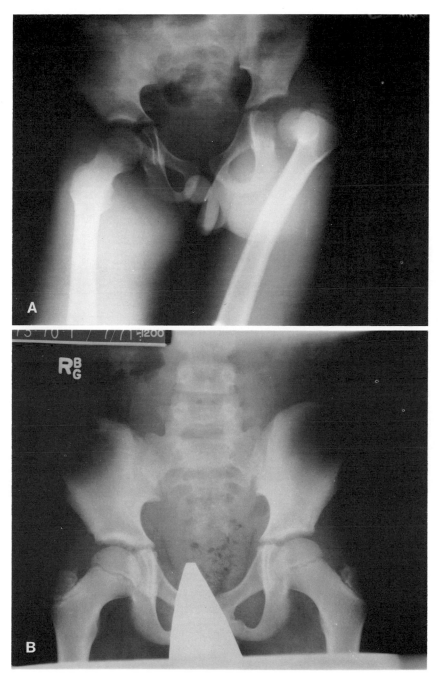

Fig. 5.26 *A*, this 7-year-old male dislocated his left hip in falling off a bicycle, sustaining a type I injury. Reduction was accomplished 2 hours after injury with iv Demerol by the Stimson maneuver. Buck's traction was used for 13 days then full weight-bearing by the 3rd week. *B*, the result after 5 years is excellent. There are no hip complaints and the range of motion is normal. The roentgenogram of the left hip is normal.

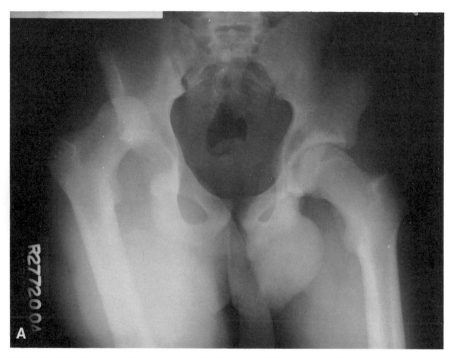

Fig. 5.27 *A*, this 14-year-old male sustained a type I dislocation. He was a passenger on a motorcycle that collided with an automobile. The result 29 months later is considered good although there are changes attributed to traumatic arthritis. Roentgenogram reveals a posterior dislocation of the right hip without fracture.

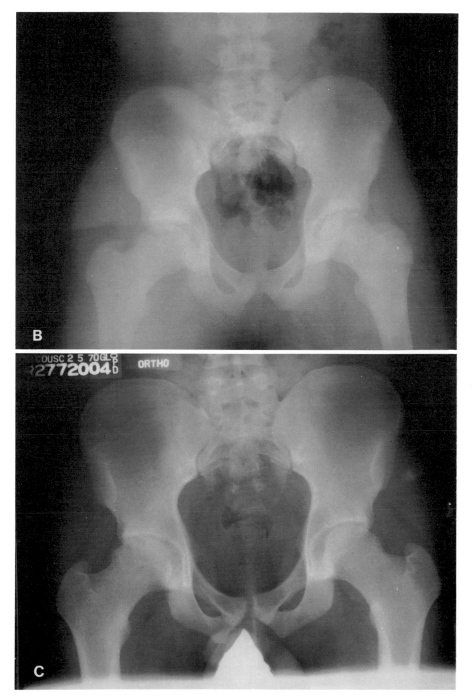

Fig. 5.27 *B*, the dislocation was reduced closed the day of injury under a general anesthesic. Traction was maintained for 3 weeks and the patient walked in 10 weeks. There is a suggestion of widening of the right hip joint. *C*, at 29 months later the result is rated good although there is beginning spur formation at the superior margin of the head-neck junction.

believes coxa magna is related to avascular necrosis, the cause being an increase in the blood supply. Powers and Bach[87] recently described coxa magna, but none of the hips involved had traumatic dislocations.

It is interesting to follow the progression of coxa magna in our case (Fig. 5.13A–H), after a closed reduction. The roentgenograms revealed a nonconcentric reduction. However, an arthrotomy was not performed until 7 days after his injury. At surgery it was found that the femoral head had buttonholed through the capsule with pressure over one-half of the articular cartilage. At the 4-month follow-up the hip appeared to be normal. The patient did not return to the clinic until 2 years after his injury, at which time the involved hip revealed a coxa magna. The patient walked without a limp and had no complaints. At 3 years the coxa magna was more evident. The patient stated he had constant hip pain and had minimal restriction of hip motion. The last clinic visit was 66 months after injury. At this time there was also a coxa valgus deformity with approximately ½ inch of overgrowth of the involved lower extremity. The patient tires easily after activities and there is approximately 25% limitation of hip motion (Fig. 5.13A–H).

The method of reduction and type of aftercare will be discussed in Chapters 6 and 7.

CHAPTER
6

TYPE OF AFTERCARE

Treatment of traumatic dislocations depends upon the type of dislocation and procedure of reduction that has been followed. The most common method of immobilization used at the Medical Center is the application of a balanced skeletal traction with a pin through the upper tibia, or skin traction (Russell's or Buck's). A spica cast may be necessary at times because of the occurrence of associated injuries to the lower extremity. Although Brav[9] advocates keeping the hip in complete extension after reduction, the policy at this institution is to keep the hip in about 20° to 30° of flexion. This is more comfortable for the patient and to date we have had no hip redislocate following this method of traction immobilization.

Traction after reduction of a fracture-dislocation should be maintained as long as it takes to unite a fracture of the acetabular rim to the acetabulum, or the combination of fractured acetabular rim and floor in a type IV dislocation. This may take as long as 6 to 8 weeks for an acetabular fracture to unite. Roentgenograms should determine the ultimate length of time for continuation of traction.

In simple anterior and posterior type I dislocations, both in children and adults, it takes a minimum of 3 to 4 weeks for the torn capsule to heal. Therefore, I feel that amount of time should be sufficient for traction. As stated previously, one-third of our patients with simple dislocations walked by the end of the 1st month and, as stated by Trueta,[102] the best way to prevent osteoporosis is by increased muscle action and the best means is by early weight-bearing.

I consider traction a better method of treatment after reduction of a dislocation than application of a spica cast, although some of the children have been sent home with spica casts applied after a few weeks of hospitalization in traction. With traction, physical therapy can be started early and this muscle action is beneficial in continuing the stresses and strains necessary in bone to prevent osteoporosis.

Since there is a positive pressure relationship between the head and acetabulum, a distracting pull will keep some of this pressure away. This would be beneficial in those dislocations in which the femoral head has suffered some injury such as excoriations, depressions, and minute fractures in the femoral head.

After traction is discontinued weight-bearing may be started with the use of crutches, provided there is no pain or muscle spasm. Start with 25% of full weight-bearing and gradually progress to full weight-bearing until the crutches can be discarded. Exercises, both active and passive, are a necessary part of therapy.

Roentgenograms should be taken immediately after closed or open reductions. These films should include both an anteroposterior and lateral view of both hips so as to check and compare the joint spaces. A widening of the cartilaginous space of the involved hip should place the orthopaedist on the alert either to an incomplete reduction, or to the probability of loose fragments in the hip joint, or to the possibility that a screw used for the fixation of an acetabular fracture may have penetrated the femoral head. Immediate measures should be undertaken to correct these conditions.

A widened joint space in a type I dislocation in children and adults suggests soft tissue intervention such as capsular invagination into the hip joint (two cases), or to a detached acetabular labrum that prevented concentric reduction (three cases), or to buttonholing of the femoral head through the capsule (one case).

Follow-up on patients who have had dislocations of their hips should be a minimum of 5 years even though the results in the majority of patients will not change after the 1st year following reduction. Three patients improved from fair to good after the first 12 months.

Of the 75 hips followed for more than 10 years, 11 had begun to show early signs of traumatic arthritis, including minimum narrowing of the cartilage space and spur formation at the junction of the femoral head and neck. Two of these hips (type V injuries) which had been rated good at 15 months and 5 years after injury, respectively, were reclassified as poor. Two type I injuries also classified as a good result at 5 years and 9 years, respectively, were reclassified as a poor result 12 years later and as a fair result 16 years after injury.

Warnings should be given the patient regarding certain signs and symptoms that may be a prelude to traumatic arthritis or avascular necrosis. Any aching in the knee or hip, inability to sit for more than 2 hours because of stiffness in the hip, occasional "giving way" feeling of the knee or hip, or a limp after walking should be a warning to the patient that his hip is not normal.

Roentgenograms should be taken at least every 3 months during the 1st year, then at 6-month intervals. Both hips should be filmed for comparison, noting whether there is narrowing of the involved hip joint or beginning spur formation at the junction of the femoral head and neck. These are early signs of traumatic arthritis. Variations in densities with minimal depression over the weight-bearing portion of the femoral head may be indicative of early avascular necrosis.

Clinical examination of the patient is essential. Moderate restriction of hip motion with reflex spasm at the extremes of motion are important. Atrophy of the involved thigh is very significant as to hip pathology, although the patient may also have had an ipsilateral injury to the knee.

CHAPTER
7

OPERATIVE METHOD

The surgical approach used in the majority of open reductions was the same as that described by Griswold and Herd[39] in 1929 and later used by King and Richards[60] (Fig. 7.1A–F). The operation is done under endotracheal anesthesia with the patient placed in a prone position. The incision extends from the posterior-superior iliac spine outward and downward to the region of the greater trochanter. For more adequate exposure the incision can be extended further laterally through the aponeurosis of the gluteus maximus and tensor fascia lata muscles. Very little bleeding is encountered if the gluteus maximus muscle is split with blunt dissection rather than incised with a sharp instrument. The areolar and fatty tissue in the region of the peritrochanteric bursa is removed. Before incision of the short rotator muscles at their attachments to the trochanteric fossa, the sciatic nerve must be identified and retracted. After incision of the short rotator muscles—mainly the piriformis, the gemelli, and the obturator internus and obturator externus—the hip joint can be adequately visualized. If further exposure is necessary the gluteus medius is divided at its attachment to the greater trochanter. This surgical approach affords excellent exposure of the hip joint and makes it possible with the hip dislocated to visualize the whole acetabulum and to remove loose fragments. Similarly, after reduction the hip joint can be stabilized by fixing the fractured posterior acetabular rim with one or more screws if necessary (see Procedures 7.1–7.6).

Other approaches used were the Gibson posterolateral exposure of the hip joint and Moore's southern approach to the hip. I have had no experience with the medial approach to the hip joint first described by Ludloff in 1913. This was used by Kelly and Yarbrough[58] for their operative approach to type V fracture-dislocations for either fixation or removal of avulsed head fragments.

The anterior iliofemoral approach of Smith-Peterson was the usual one used in our series for the anterior approaches (Procedure 7.7).

Eleven open reductions, both primary and secondary, were done through an anterior approach for posterior dislocations; two for type II, three for type IV, and six for type V lesions. In these 11 hips the result was fair in one type V hip and poor in two type III, three type IV, and four type V hips. In the remaining type V case, not included in the final statistics, the result was not known because of insufficient follow-up (Procedures 7.8–7.10).

It is likely that most, if not all, of the blood supply to the hip joint is damaged when a posterior dislocation occurs. A surgical procedure that embarrasses whatever anterior blood supply remains is therefore inadvisable. In performing the anterior iliofemoral approach to the hip, the ascending branch of the lateral femoral circumflex artery must be ligated. The capsule also must be incised to expose the femoral head. Although the number of anterior approaches made in this group is relatively small, the absence of good results in the 10 hips with adequate follow-up after this approach was used strongly suggests that it is inadvisable (Fig. 3.31A–C).

Stewart and Milford[95] reported that 75% of their open reductions on posterior dislocated hips were performed through the anterior approach. This is possibly one of the reasons their open reductions had poorer results than those treated closed.

One should consider the potentially harmful effects of surgery before an open procedure is undertaken. In this large series, one patient died of cardiac arrest during surgery; another patient with irreducible dislocation signed out against consent (he later died during surgery for a reconstructive procedure); and 12 had postoperative infections. On the other hand, comminuted fragments not visible on roentgenograms can be removed and the posterior acetabular lip in an unstable hip can be fixed only by arthrotomy and open reduction.

In the majority of the operative procedures the large acetabular fragment was usually securely fixed with screws of adequate length and size to the main portion of the posterior acetabular rim. In a few instances, nails or pins were used because

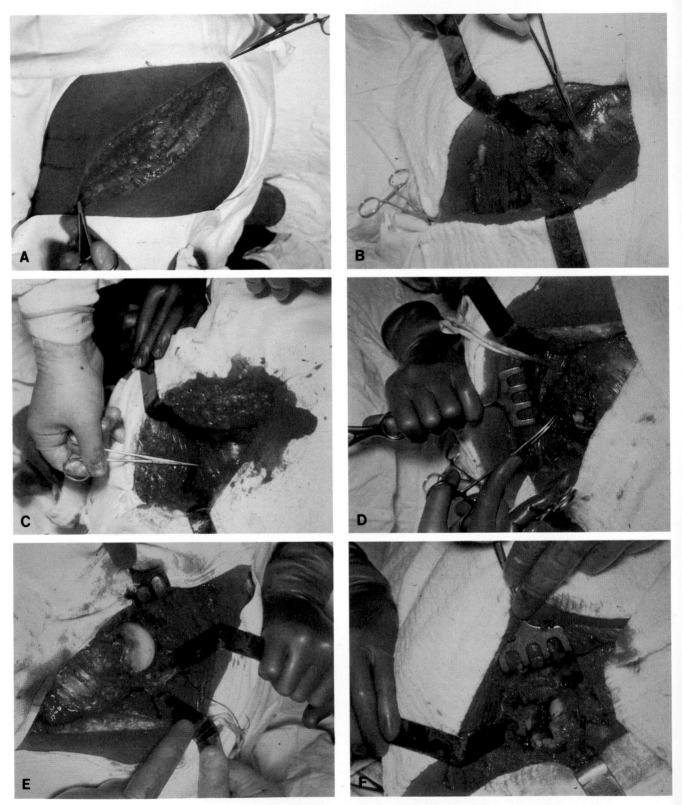

Fig. 7.1 Operative approach. *A*, prone position. Incision extends from posterior-superior iliac spine outward and downward to region of the greater trochanter. *B*, split gluteus maximus muscle with blunt dissection. The hemostat is pointing to the areolar and fatty tissue in the peritrochanteric region. *C*, the sciatic nerve is identified. *D*, the penrose drain surrounds and isolates the sciatic nerve. Observe the hemorrhage in this region. *E*, the short rotators are detached with sutures between the incisions for better approximation later. The femoral head is readily visible. *F*, after approximation of the ischium and ilium with one screw and fixation of the posterior acetabular rim with two screws, there is a large gap posteriorly because many smaller fragments had to be discarded.

the fragments were too small or too thin for screw fixation and were discarded (Fig. 7.2*A–E*). In two instances fixation of the avulsed posterior fragment was attempted by catgut sutures and in both cases the fragment later displaced with subluxation of the hip (Fig. 3.20*A–E*). One should measure for size and length of the screw used for immobilization of the posterior rim fragment. There were two hips in which the acetabular rim fragment displaced after surgery with subluxation of the hip because the screw was not long enough to secure adequate fixation.

In the type V dislocations the usual procedure was to discard the avulsed fracture off the posterior-inferior portion of the femoral head. Two patients had the avulsed head fragment reattached to the main portion of the head by screw fixation. However, one of these became infected and in the other the result was unknown because of insufficient follow-up.

One should always take check roentgenograms of the hip prior to closure to determine, first, whether there were loose fragments left in the hip joint, and second, whether the screw used for fixation penetrated the femoral head, as occurred in one of our cases (Figs. 3.23*A–E* and 3.25*A–C*).

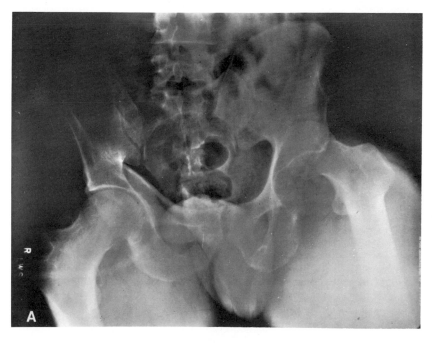

Fig. 7.2 *A*, a 36-year-old male injured in an auto vs. auto accident sustained this type III posterior dislocation of the right hip. A closed reduction was followed 2 days later by an open procedure. Four years later the result is poor with avascular necrosis. *A*, roentgenogram reveals posterior dislocation of right hip with multiple fragments.

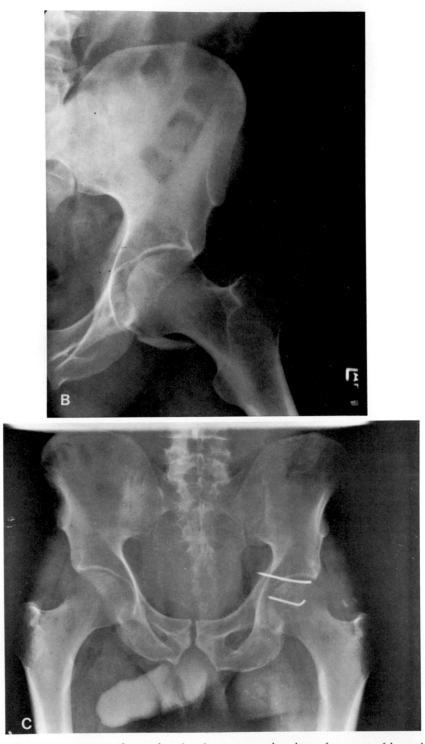

Fig. 7.2 *B*, roentgenogram after a closed reduction reveals a large fragment of bone lying inferiorly within the joint space. *C*, roentgenogram taken after surgery. The hip was redislocated and many loose fragments of bone and debris were removed from the hip joint. The acetabular labrum was detached posteriorly. There was a small fracture through the anterior superior portion of the femoral head involving the cartilage and subchrondral bone. Two large Steinmann pins were used to transfix the large posterior acetabular rim. Attempts to use screw fixation were unsuccessful.

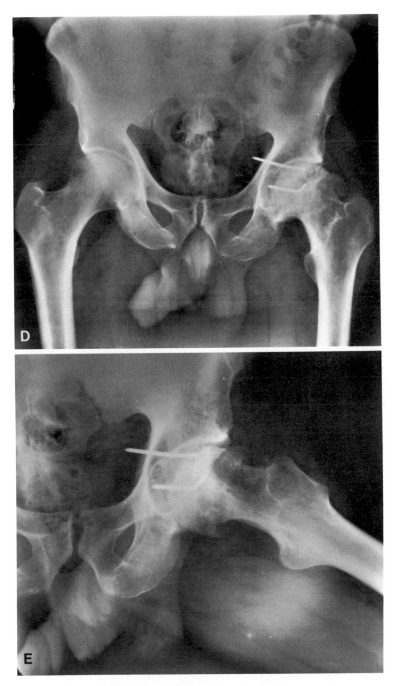

Fig. 7.2 *D* and *E*, roentgenograms taken at follow-up reveal avascular necrosis with areas of increased densities, irregularities, and supr formation of the femoral head. The superior Steinmann pin has penetrated slightly into the pelvis. The patient had moderate limitation of hip motion with pain on weight-bearing. He stated his hip was painful 2 months after his surgery. Reconstructive surgery is being considered.

PROCEDURE

Operator: H. C. Epstein, M.D.

Preoperative Diagnosis: Transcervical fracture of left femur with posterior
dislocation of the head of the left femur

Procedure 7.1:

The left hip was prepared and draped in the usual fashion with the patient prone on the
operating table. An incision was made across the left buttock extending across the region
of the posterior-superior iliac spine to the greater trochanter. Incision was carried down
through the fascia to expose the gluteus maximus muscle. By blunt dissection, the fibers
of the gluteus maximus were spread apart, revealing the rotator cuff and the gluteus
medius. The sciatic nerve was then identified and retracted from the operative area. The
rotator cuff and gluteus medius were then detached from their insertions. Exploration of
the wound revealed several loose fragments in the hip joint which were removed. It was
found that there was some attachment from the fracture head of the femur and the neck
and it was felt that reposition of the head offered a chance for possible healing. With great
difficulty, it was possible to relocate the head of the femur into the hip joint. Two Austin
Moore pins were then inserted into the neck of the femur across the fracture site to the
head of the femur. A check film revealed these pins to be of satisfactory length and
satisfactory position. The fracture site was felt fairly stable on passive motion. The wound
was then closed with reattachment of the rotator cuff and gluteus medius and suture of
the fascia and skin. Pressure dressing was applied and the patient was placed in Russell's
traction. Condition was considered satisfactory.

Operator: H. C. Epstein, M.D.

Preoperative Diagnosis: Fracture-dislocation, neck of the left femur, with
previous internal fixation with two Moore pins

Procedure 7.2:

After routine preparation and draping, the distal two-thirds of the original scar was
excised and a 6-inch incision over the greater trochanter along the lateral site of the femur
was made and carried down to the fascia lata; the latter was incised and freed-up. The
fascia over the vastus lateralis was incised; the intertrochanteric insertion of the latter's
muscle was split transversely and the subtrochanteric attachment was split longitudinally
for a distance of 3 inches and elevated, exposing the previously placed ends of the Moore
pins which were fixed in scar tissue. A $\frac{3}{8}$-inch-diameter drill hole was placed just below the
flare of the greater trochanter, paralleling the original pins and carried well into the head
of the femur, in preparing a site for a dowel bone graft. Next, a 2-inch incision was made
over the left anterior-superior crest of the ilium. The periosteum was elevated. Bleeding
was controlled with packs, and with an osteotome a $1\frac{1}{2}$-inch $\times$ $\frac{3}{8}$ inch sliver of outer table
bone graft and its cancellous bone were removed. Three such bone graft pieces were
selected and driven into the previously prepared femoral tract. These were driven until
firm, one bending the other. A Moore pin was now introduced paralleling the bone graft
site and carried well into the head. The aforementioned protruding Moore pin was
extracted $\frac{1}{2}$ inch, but not tightened, and it was cut off appropriately; x-ray at this time
showed the pins to be in adequate position and the fracture site reduced. The third Moore
pin was cut off. The fascia of the vastus lateralis was closed using No. 0 chromic, as was
the fascia lata with a running locked stitch. Subcutaneous tissue was closed using interrupted No. 000 chromic, and the skin was closed with No. 35 wire vertical mattress running
suture. The periosteum over the iliac bone site was closed using No. 00 chromic, the
subcutaneous tissues with the same running suture, and the skin with No. 34 vertical
mattress interrupted sutures. The patient lost approximately 700 ml of blood and appeared
to tolerate surgery well.

Operator: H. C. Epstein, M.D.

Preoperative Diagnosis: Posterior dislocation of left hip with fragmented head of femur and acetabulum

Procedure 7.3:

Under nitrous oxide anesthesia with the patient lying in the prone position, an incision was made, curvilinear in fashion, extending from just below the inferior-posterior spine of the ilium lateralward over the posterolateral aspect of the buttock down to and opposite to the greater trochanter. The skin incision extended down to the superficial fascia which, after being cut, revealed the gluteus maximus and gluteus medius musculature. By blunt dissection through the cleavage of the muscle planes the piriformis, gemellus superior, and gemellus inferior muscles were identified. Further blunt dissection more medialward revealed the sciatic nerve. After the sciatic nerve was identified, isolated, and retracted, No. 1 silks were inserted in the tendinous insertion of the piriformis muscle and the piriformis muscle was cut and retracted over the sciatic nerve. Another No. 1 silk was inserted in the stump of the piriformis tendon and Kelly applied to this suture. The gemellus superior and inferior were treated likewise and were cut at their insertions and retracted, revealing the capsule of the femoral neck and head. The capsule was torn by virtue of the traumatic impact of the dislocation. The rim of the acetabulum was identified, and by retracting the overlying structures the examining finger could be placed in the acetabulum and the fragments felt. With the examining finger the large fragment was delivered from the acetabulum with moderate difficulty and ligamentum teres was incised and fragment removed. On further palpation a smaller fragment was felt and removed with the examining finger. With the assistant holding the distal end of the femur (which also had a supracondylar fracture and had been previously splinted) to facilitate movement during the surgery with a traction force and with the operator manipulating the hip joint, the head of the femur was delivered into the acetabulum. The range of motion was checked and the joint was found to be in good position. The surgical incision was then closed by removing the Penrose drain from the sciatic nerve, permitting it to retract into its previous position, after which the gemellus superior and inferior and the piriformis were reattached by means of previously inserted sutures, being made fast from the proximal to the distal and from the distal to the proximal ends of the musculature. A few interrupted sutures were inserted to approximate the muscles which had been bluntly separated, after which the fascia was closed with No. 00 interrupted chromic sutures. The overlying skin was then closed with No. 35 stainless steel wire continuous sutures. Bandages were applied. Patient was placed in a femur bed with Hodgen-Pearson suspension traction and was sent to the ward in fair condition.

Operator: H. C. Epstein, M.D.

Preoperative Diagnosis: Posterior dislocation of the right hip with a fracture of the posterior acetabulum

Procedure 7.4:

Under endotracheal anesthesia and with the patient in prone position, a 12-inch incision was made over the right buttock beginning approximately 2 inches distal to the posterior-superior iliac spin and running in a slightly curved manner down over the posterior aspect of the greater trochanter and distally along the shaft of the femur approximately 4 inches. This was developed down to the fascia of the gluteus maximus, which was then split by blunt dissection through the length of the incision, the incision being extended in a distal portion of the wound by incision of the fascia lata. By sharp and blunt dissection, the adipose tissue underlying the gluteus maximus was removed, exposing the sciatic nerve, around which an umbilical tape was placed, retracting the sciatic nerve then medially. A figure-of-8 No. 2 silk suture was then placed into the short external rotator along its insertion into the greater trochanter and just proximal to this. The muscles were incised between the sutures and the medial portions were retracted so as to expose the femoral head and acetabulum. The femoral head was then reduced. One fragment was removed and the remaining fragment was transfixed to the posterior acetabulum rim by a single transfixing screw. The hip then appeared to be stable. The short rotators were reattached by means of previously placed sutures. The fascia of the gluteus maximus was closed with No. 00 chromic interrupted suture; the fascia lata, with No. 0 chromic interrupted sutures; and skin, with No. 34 wire vertical mattress interrupted sutures. The patient was placed in Russell's traction.

Operator: H. C. Epstein, M.D.

Preoperative Diagnosis: Fracture-dislocation, posterior left hip, with large fragment off the posterior superior rim

Procedure 7.5:

Under spinal anesthesia, a Kocher posterior approach was made, starting at the posterior-superior spine and curving the incision downward to the base of the greater trochanter and laterally 1½ inches. Skin was toweled off and the incision then proceeded through the fascia covering the gluteus maximus. Then with finger dissection, the gluteus maximus fibers were split 1 inch below the posterior-superior spine of the ilium. This exposed the areolar tissue, fatty tissue covering the short rotator muscles. By gentle sharp dissection the areolar tissue and fat were removed. This brought the short rotator muscles into view. The piriformis muscle was identified; it was intact and it was retracted upward. The sciatic nerve was isolated and retracted with a linen cloth. The short rotator muscles remaining were severed near the base of the greater trochanter, first placing chromic No. 2 sutures proximal and distal to the severance. The short rotator muscle was then retracted medially—this exposed the capsule well. There was sufficient rent in the capsule so that it was not necessary to elongate the incision. All visible bleeders were ligated with No. 00 chromic. There was considerable attachment of the avulsed fragment of the acetabular rim which included the posterior portion of the capsule. The fragments were curetted out and bled easily, signifying a good blood supply. The fragment was then replaced anatomically and held in position with one Kirschner wire directed upward to the thick portion of the acetabulum. A 1½-inch screw was then inserted and this held the fragments in good position and appeared strong. Internal and external rotation of the head of the femur was done easily without any interference. There were no visible bony fragments in the hip joint. The torn capsule was then approximated with No. 0 chromic. Short rotator muscles were approximated with the sutures that had already been placed. The sciatic nerve was put in position. Fascia was closed—the fascia closed over the gluteus maximus—then approximated, and the superficial fascia and skin were closed. There was no evidence of bleeding.

Operator: H. C. Epstein, M.D.

Preoperative Diagnosis: Dislocation of the left hip, fracture of the left acetabulum, and free bony particles within the hip joint

Procedure 7.6:

After general anesthesia and pHisoHex skin preparation, the patient was placed in a prone position with one sandbag under the left hip. Skin incision was made extending to a point approximately 1 cm lateral and inferior to the posterior-inferior iliac spine, to the crest of the greater trochanter, and approximately 2 cm down the shaft of the femur. Dissection was carried down to the deep fascia; bleeders were either tied with No. 00 plain, or hemostasis was obtained with cautery. The interval between the posterior fibers of the gluteus maximus was then located and split distally in the line with the incision. A large hematoma was found directly posterior to the gluteus maximus and cleaned away. Dissection was then carried down to the adipose tissue to the trochanteric fossa and then posteriorly until the sciatic nerve was identified. Sciatic nerve was secured with a loop of Penrose drain and gently retracted posteriorly and medially. The tendinous insertion of external rotators of the hip was then cut, after the proximal and distal ends of these muscles had been secured with No. 0 silk figure-of-8 sutures. At this point, a definite rent in the posterior capsule was noted. Signs of trauma were present about the joint, such as thrombosed veins and blood vessels and a few small bony particles. In addition, a large bony fragment, much greater in dimensions than had been suspected by x-ray, was found present through the sizable defect in the posterior acetabulum which would have made a stable hip joint impossible. The hip was then dislocated with moderate difficulty due to inability to obtain adequate flexion of the thigh and the presence of intact ligamentum teres which had to be sacrificed. Digital palpation of the acetabular cavity revealed the presence of three or four medium- to small-sized free bony particles, which were carefully removed. The large fragmented acetabulum was then replaced in approximately anatomical position after reduction of the dislocation of the hip, and a single screw was driven through this fragment into the ilium. Adequate and stable reduction of the fracture and of the hip was then found to be present. The tendons of the external rotators were repaired and tied in place with previously described sutures. The deep fascia was repaired with No. 0 chromic continuous; subcutaneous tissues were repaired with No. 00 chromic interrupted; and skin was closed with No. 34 wire. Patient left the operating room in good condition after a check film had been taken which showed satisfactory position of hip, fracture, and screw.

Operator: H. C. Epstein, M.D.

Preoperative Diagnosis: Anterior dislocation of the left femur, compound fracture of the mandible with multiple lacerations

Procedure 7.7:

There was found to be a medial anterior dislocation of the femur with a fracture of the femoral head, exposing the anterior articular cortex. The femoral head was incarcerated in the tear in the joint capsule anteriorly and inferiorly. With the patient under general anesthesia, the skin overlying the hip was prepared with ether, alcohol, and tincture of QAA and draped in the routine manner. An anterior approach to the hip was made in the following manner: The skin incision was started parallel to the iliac crest, extending about 4 inches to the anterosuperior iliac spine, then distally and slightly laterally on the leg for a distance of approximately 4 inches. This was carried down through the fascia to the iliac crest. The lateral femoral cutaneous nerve was identified and retracted medially. The space between the rectus femoris and the tensor fascia lata was then entered. The tensor fascia lata and the gluteus medius were removed from the iliac crest for a distance approximately 3½ to 4 inches. The lateral femoral circumflex artery was clamped and ligated with No. 0 chromic ties. The remaining bleeders were clamped and hemostasis was achieved using the Bovie. Using blunt and sharp dissection, exposure was carried down to the level of the acetabulum. The joint capsule was identified and opened in the direction of its fibers, the ligament of Bigelow being incised transversely. The femoral head was then reduced with great difficulty. The large, loose fragment from the anterior surface of the femoral head was removed. There seemed to be considerable articular weight-bearing surface left intact. The ligamentum teres was noted to be torn. There was no bleeding from the stump of the teres. The joint was cleaned out prior to reduction of the hip. The capsule was then closed with figure-of-8 No. 0 chromic suture. The vastus lateralis, which had been excised, was repaired. The tensor fascia lata and the gluteus medius were reattached to their origins from the iliac crest with interrupted No. 0 chromic sutures. The wound was irrigated thoroughly with normal saline and neomycin. The subcutaneous tissue was closed with interrupted No. 000 plain catgut sutures and the skin was closed with interrupted No. 32 wire. Postoperatively, the patient was immobilized on a Hodgen-Pearson suspension in a femur bed. The estimated blood loss was 450 ml. No drains were used. Sponge and needle counts were reported as correct at the end of the procedure.

Operator: H. C. Epstein, M.D.

Preoperative Diagnosis: Fracture of the head of the left femur with *anterior* and distal displacement of the proximal fragment

Procedure 7.8:

Open reduction of left hip joint and excision of proximal fragment: Under adequate general anesthesia a 6-inch incision was made over the anterior aspect of the left hip beginning just distal to the anterosuperior iliac spine and extending downward medial to the border of the tensor fascia lata muscle. The interval between this muscle and the rectus femoris was found and the wound was carried down to the hip joint by blunt dissection. The branches of the circumflex iliac artery and lateral femoral circumflex artery were clamped and ligated. The reflected head of the rectus femoris was detached from its origin, following which the capsule of the hip joint was opened with T-shaped incision. This gave a good view of the fracture site. It was considered impossible to fix the fracture in a reduced position and maintain reduction, therefore the proximal fragment to which was attached the ligamentum teres was excised after sectioning this ligament. The capsule was repaired with No. 0 chromic catgut and the wound was closed in layers with No. 00 chromic to the fascia, No. 000 plain to subcutaneous, and No. 35 wire to the skin. Dry sterile pressure dressing was applied and patient left surgery in good condition.

Operator: H. C. Epstein, M.D.

Preoperative Diagnosis: Dislocation of right hip, reduced with fracture of the inferior portion of the head of the left femur

Procedure 7.9:

Under satisfactory nitrous oxide and Trilene anesthesia, the right hip was prepared and draped in the usual fashion. An incision was made over the anterior aspect of the iliac crest and extended 5 inches distal to the inferior-superior iliac spine. Incision was carried down to the deep fascia, and bleeders were clamped and cauterized. The deep fascia was incised. The origin of the tensor fascia lata muscle was incised and reflected downward. The lateral femoral cutaneous nerve was identified and preserved by retracting medially with a Penrose drain. The plane between the tensor fascia lata muscle and the sartorius and rectus femoris muscles was found and dissected. The ascending branch of the lateral femoral circumflex artery was identified, clamped, and tied with No. 00 chromic sutures. The capsule of the joint was exposed and opened with a longitudinal incision. A 2 × 2 × 3 cm fragment from the anterior aspect of the head of the femur was identified and found to be rotated 180°. The fracture surface was in contact with the articular surface of the acetabulum. The fragment was dissected free and removed. The capsule was closed with interrupted No. 0 chromic interrupted sutures; the fascia was closed with interrupted No. 00 chromic sutures; subcutaneous tissue was approximated with No. 000 plain interrupted sutures; and the skin was closed with a running locked suture of No. 35 wire.

Operator: H. C. Epstein, M.D.

Preoperative Diagnosis: Posterior dislocated left hip with large fragment avulsed off the posterosuperior acetabular rim

Procedure 7.10:

Reduction, replacement of avulsed fragment with one screw: Under spinal anesthesia, a posterior approach was made through the skin from the posterosuperior iliac spine curving downward to the base of the trochanter. Skin was then toweled off; incision was made, and proceeded 1 inch below the posterior-superior spine through the muscle of the gluteus maximus. Fibers were separated bluntly in line with its direction. There was a large subcutaneous hematoma with bleeding encountered as the gluteus maximus was opened. The areolar fatty tissue was then removed and the short rotator muscles were exposed. The piriformis and the inferior and superior gemellus and obturator internus were then severed just before their attachment to the trochanter. The posterior capsule was found to be completely frayed and the head of the femur was subluxated posteriorly. A large fragment of bone off the superoposterior rim of the acetabulum, measuring approximately 4 × 2½ cm was found displaced laterally with the acetabular margin rotated through an arc of 180°. There was some attachment of the piriformis to this fragment. The hip was dislocated and a large fragment of bone measuring ½ × ¼ inches was found in the hip joint. The posterior portion of the glenoid labrum was also avulsed and the posterior capsule was completely torn with some fragments into the hip joint. This was removed also. The head of the femur was then reduced in the acetabulum. An avulsed portion was put in its proper place and held by one long screw. This seemed to hold the head of the femur securely in the acetabulum although instability of the posterior capsule was found. The short rotator muscles were then repaired using No. 1 silk and the fascia, muscle, and skin were closed in layers. Because of the glenoid labrum, which was so frayed it could not be repaired, and the complete tearing of the posterior capsule, it is possible that this hip may be unstable.

Operator: H. C. Epstein, M.D.

Preoperative Diagnosis: Bony fragment of right posterior inferior acetabulum

Procedure 7.11:

Open reduction of right hip posteriorly; removal of loose fragment: Patient had an open reduction of the left upper third of the femur done 3 weeks previously. It was found at surgery that the patient was unable to internally rotate the right hip. X-ray taken revealed bone block in the posterior-inferior surface of the acetabulum measuring approximately 1 × ½ inch by x-ray. Condition did not warrant early intervention. After routine surgical preparation of the skin, a posterior approach was made in the region of the posterior-inferior superior iliac spine down to the center of the trochanteric fossa. Skin was toweled off. Incision was extended into the fascia of the gluteus maximus. With finger dissection the gluteus maximus was opened in the line of its fibers. Two small bleeders were ligated. The sciatic nerve was identified and retracted with Penrose drain. The short rotators including the obturator internus and two gemelli were severed ½ inch from the attachment to the greater trochanter. On reflecting the short rotators medially, it was found there was a large rent in the inferior capsule measuring at least 2 inches in length and running parallel to the neck. There was a subcutaneous hematoma organization in the region of the capsule. The bony fragment was then visualized lying partly outside and partly inside the capsule. This was removed by sharp dissection and found to measure 1 × ¾ inches. A portion of the articular cortex of the acetabulum was visible. After removal of this fragment, the hip joint moved freely both on internal and external rotation. The hip joint was irrigated with saline. There was no evidence of damage to the head of the femur although the head was not dislocated. The short rotators were then sutured to the insertion and the muscles, fascia, and skin were repaired in layers. There was no external bleeding. Postoperative condition of patient was good.

Operator: H. C. Epstein, M.D.

Preoperative Diagnosis: Posterior dislocation of right hip, with comminuted fracture, posterior rim of right acetabulum

Procedure 7.12:

Open reduction, right hip dislocation, with removal of loose fragment: Under general anesthesia and with the patient in the prone position, an incision was made over the right buttocks extending from the posterior-superior spine driving slightly lateralward down over the trochanter and extending 2 inches below the greater trochanter on the lateral femur. By blunt dissection the fibers of the gluteus maximus muscle was split, the areolar tissue beneath this axis was carefully cleaned out, and the capsule and the femoral head were identified. The sciatic nerve was isolated, found to be intact, and carefully retracted by Penrose drain. A small loose fragment was then removed entirely; the head was relocated to the acetabulum which had been palpated before reduction and found to be a little rough from the acetabular fracture. No further fragments were identified. There was some scarring of the articular surface of the femoral head (like scratch marks). Following reduction, the large fragment was relocated anatomically and fixed with one screw fixation. Following this, the motion in the femoral head was free without grating. External rotators were reattached with No. 1 silk sutures. The gluteus maximus was sutured with No. 00 chromic, subcutaneous with No. 000 chromic, and skin with No. 35 wire sutures.

Operator: H. C. Epstein, M.D.

Preoperative Diagnosis: Posterosuperior dislocation, right femur, with fragmentation on the posterior rim of the acetabulum

Procedure 7.13:

Open reduction, posterior approach, removal of bone chips: The patient was positioned on his stomach with the right pelvis slightly elevated. Chest rolls were used. The patient was prepared and draped, exposing the right buttock. A stockinette was used to cover the exposed area. A modified type of Gibson incision was used, distally along the shaft from the greater trochanter to the posterosuperior spine for 6 inches. This was carried down through the subcutaneous tissue to the underlying fascia and gluteus maximus. An incision was made in the fascia, and the fibers of the gluteus maximus were separated by finger dissection in the line of their axis. The underlying gluteus medius was identified, and a row of No. 1 silk sutures placed at its insertion ½ inch apart. An incision was made between the two sutures and the muscle was reflected. Underlying gluteus minimus was likewise identified and retracted. The piriformis and superior gemellus were likewise identified and retracted. This permitted palpation of the joint space and evaluation of the area without further detachment of the short rotator muscle. The above-described largest fragment, because it was too thin to screw despite its large surface area, was removed and sent to pathology as a specimen, as were the other smaller chips. The joint was inspected and the entire capsule was found to lie within the joint space. Little bits of minute bone gravel were removed from the head. The head had three or four superficial excoriations presumably where it had struck the rim of the acetabulum. These were believed to be minor injuries. The capsule was removed from the joint space, irrigated with 700 ml of sterile saline, the last 20 ml of which contained 1 g of neomycin. With manipulation and a bone skid, the femur was reduced; the soft musculature was allowed to fall in place. The superior gemellus, the piriformis, and the gluteus minimus and medius were reattached with No. 1 silk suture—in that sequence. No. 0 chromic interrupted sutures were used to reinforce the repair. The gluteus maximus fibers were allowed to fall in place. Overlying fascia was sutured with running No. 0 chromic, subcutaneous tissue with interrupted No. 00 chromic, and skin with running No. 34 suture. Vaseline gauze dry sterile dressing was applied; patient's leg was held in abduction during entire procedure after reduction and was placed in traction in abduction with 5 lb of Buck's traction. Patient lost approximately 350 ml of blood. He appeared to tolerate the procedure well.

Operator: H. C. Epstein, M.D.

Preoperative Diagnosis: Posterior fracture-dislocation of left hip, 14-year-old child

Procedure 7.14:

Open reduction, left hip: Under adequate nitrous oxide oxygen-Pentothal anesthesia, the patient was placed prone on appropriate shoulder-hip rolls, an extra pad being placed under the left hip. The left lower extremity was draped free. A posterolateral modified Gibson incision was used. The gluteus maximus was freed in part from its insertion into the tensor fascia lata and split in the area between the upper third and lower two-thirds. The sciatic nerve was isolated by blunt dissection and carefully preserved with a rubber dam drain. The short external rotators of the hip were divided between No. 0 silk sutures, and the posterior capsule and acetabulum of the hip joint were exposed, revealing the aforementioned findings. The capsule was incised longitudinally and carefully opened above and below, utilizing in part the rent through which it was protruding. The hip was dislocated and the acetabulum was profusely irrigated with sterile saline. Only two or three fragments of articular cartilage were found free in the joint. The 2 × 3 cm piece of the posterior-superior acetabular rim with its smaller attached companion piece was replaced into its bed and affixed with two screws after having replaced the head of the femur into the acetabulum. The capsule was closed with No. 0 chromic. The short rotators were tied back together with pieces of silk mentioned above. Further layer closure was attained by the use of No. 00 chromic and No. 0 chromic after hemostasis had been achieved with No. 000 plain. The skin was closed with No. 34 wire simple and vertical mattress interrupted sutures. Patient was transferred to bed in good condition in Hodgen-Pearson suspension.

CHAPTER
8

MULTIPLE INJURIES

Multiple injuries were sustained in 121 cases (Table 8.1). Not included in the statistics were 18 patients (17 adults and one child, age 15 years), who died of multiple injuries following their accidents. Forty-five of these associated injuries were in the anterior and posterior type I dislocation group.

There were nine bilateral dislocations, one bilateral anterior (Fig. 4.9A, B), one bilateral posterior (type I) (Fig. 5.1A, B) in a child, and seven bilateral with an anterior dislocation on one side and a posterior dislocation on the other side (Fig. 4.5).

Twenty-seven of the patients with multiple injuries had ipsilateral fractures of the femur. There were two in anterior dislocations, both recognized at the time of injury, with an excellent result in a child, age 13 (Fig. 4.14), and a good result in an adult. Seven dislocations occurred in type I; one, not recognized for 2 weeks, had a poor result and the other poor case, although recognized, was irreducible by closed method and an open reduction was performed 2½ months after injury because of the poor condition of the patient. Good results occurred in the three dislocations that were recognized. The results in two cases are unknown because of insufficient follow-up.

Eighteen fracture-dislocations of the hip were associated with distal fractures of the ipsilateral femur, three in the supracondylar region and 15 at the midshaft level. The results in five of these fracture-dislocations (one type II, one type III, two type IV, and one type V) were unknown because of insufficient follow-up and are not included in the final results. In the remaining 13 cases the results were good in a type II, a type III, a type IV, and a type V, and poor in a type II, in four type III cases, and in three type IV and one type V.

In the type II case in which there was a good result, the fracture in the mid-third of the femur was fixed with an intramedullary rod and the hip fracture-dislocation was reduced by closed manipulation. One day later an open reduction was performed. In the type III lesion in which the result was good, the dislocation was reduced closed at another hospital and then transferred to the Los Angeles County-University of Southern California Medical Center, where an open reduction was performed and the supracondylar fracture treated in Russell traction. In the type IV lesion with a good result a primary open reduction was performed and the femoral fracture was treated in traction. In the type V dislocation in which the result was good, the supracondylar fracture was treated in traction and the fracture-dislocation was treated by primary open reduction which was delayed 8 days because of skull fracture. In the type II lesion in which there was a poor result, the dislocation was not recognized for 9 days and the patient then refused an open reduction. In one of the four type III cases with a poor result a postoperative infection occurred after internal fixation of the shaft fracture with an intramedullary nail combined with primary open reduction of the fracture-

Table 8.1
Results: Multiple Injuries in Traumatic Dislocations of the Hip

Type	Excellent-good	Fair	Poor	Total	Percentage
Anterior	7	1	1	9	7
Children	4	2	2	8	7
Type I	16	3	9	28	23
Type II	14	5	1	20	17
Type III	11	10	11	32	26
Type IV	2	3	7	12	10
Type V	4	2	6	12	10
Total	58	26	37	121	100
Percentage	48%	21%	31%		

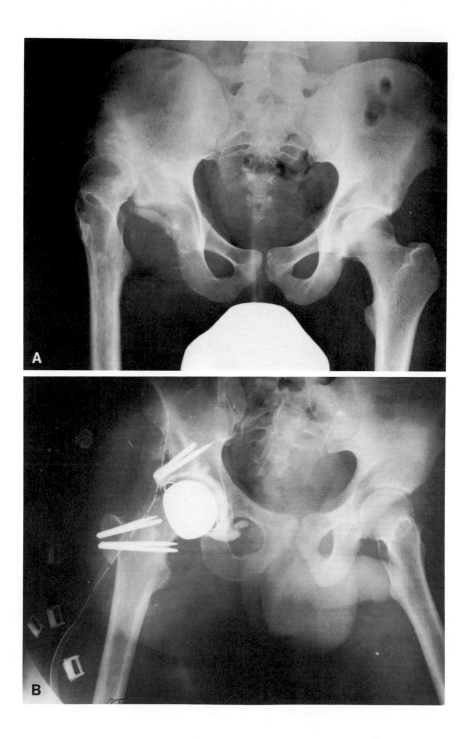

Fig. 8.1   A 26-year-old man in an automobile accident was first seen in the emergency room for a closed fracture of the right tibia and fibula. This fracture was treated in the trauma clinic. Eight months after injury he complained of a painful right hip and roentgenograms revealed a posterior dislocation, type III. A resurfacing procedure was performed one month later at another hospital. *A*, roentgenogram of the right hip 8 months after injury. *B*, roentgenogram after reconstructive surgery. The result is unknown because of insufficient follow-up.

dislocation of the hip. In two patients the dislocation was not recognized 9 and 10 days after injury, and in the last case a closed reduction was done because of the poor condition of the patient.

Two of the type IV fracture-dislocations were not recognized. One was associated with an anterior hip dislocation on the other side which was recognized while the posterior dislocation on the side of the shaft fracture was overlooked (Fig. 3.17A-C). The other, seen in a 14-year-old girl, was not recognized for approximately 2 months; attempted open reduction 10 months after injury was unsuccessful because of soft tissue contractures (Fig. 5.20). The third type IV fracture-dislocation was not reduced when closed reduction was attempted; 2 weeks after injury intramedullary fixation of the shaft fracture and open reduction of the hip was performed. Nine months after injury a total hip replacement was performed because of painful traumatic arthritis. The type V fracture-dislocation was not recognized and later had a successful hip fusion.

In the presence of a fracture of the femoral shaft or condyles, the hip injury is easily overlooked. For the past 18 years it has been a policy at the Medical Center to obtain roentgenograms of the pelvis of all patients admitted with severe injuries. Since this policy has been in effect, no dislocations of the hip with ipsilateral fracture of the femur have gone unrecognized. (In a recent type II case not included in the statistics, a 26-year-old man was treated in the emergency room for a fracture of the right tibia and fibula and not hospitalized. Eight months later the fracture-dislocation was diagnosed in the trauma clinic) (Fig. 8.1A, B).

Treatment of traumatic dislocations of the hip with ipsilateral fractures of the femur has been discussed by many orthopaedists.[9, 16, 17, 106, 111]

The author agrees with Watson-Jones[108] that the fracture should first be reduced and immobilized by internal fixation before the hip is reduced. In a majority of cases this was the procedure used. Three of the six ipsilateral fractures of the femur treated by closed reduction were supracondylar.

Nine dislocations of the hip, other than those with ipsilateral fractured femurs, went unrecognized for from 1 month to 6 months. Two occurred in outside hospitals, seven were in type III dislocations, one in a type V dislocation, and the other in an anterior dislocation. All had multiple injuries. Two of the hips were later fused with good results. Two had cup arthroplasties. One, good for 12 years later, because of pain had a total hip implant with a good result. In the other cup arthroplasty the hip dislocated 1 month after surgery but the patient refused a further procedure. A Whitman reconstruction failed in one case and in the other four cases the hips were left unreduced.

CHAPTER
9

COMPLICATIONS

It may be difficult to differentiate avascular necrosis and severe traumatic arthritis, especially when a single roentgenogram is reviewed some time after injury. Many authors believe that the cause of avascular necrosis is the tearing of some blood vessels and thrombosis of others at the time of injury and treatment (Fig. 3.24*A, B*). Urist[105] believes thrombosis of the blood vessels at the retinacula of Weitbrecht and the posterior reflected capsule of the hip joint may be the cause of avascular necrosis. Other causes for this serious complication have been suggested. Steward and Milford[95] believe that a strong force acting on the femoral head may cause molecular changes resulting in avascular necrosis of bone. Sledge[93a] believes a strong force acting on the femoral head on impact may result in death of both chondrocytes and osteocytes. Garden[33] suggested that malreduction causing incongruity of the hip joint following subcapital fracture is associated with a segmental collapse of the femoral head. I have noted the roentgenographic findings of avascular necrosis in the early stage to be a depression of the subchondral bone of the femoral head with areas of increased and decreased densities, usually with a preserved joint space (Fig. 3.18*A–C*). Later changes are a defect with irregularity and collapse of the femoral head with more areas of changes in density. Only the femoral head is involved (Figs. 3.21*A–C*; 5.19*A–D*; 5.21*A–C*). More advanced changes may be difficult to differentiate from the severe changes in traumatic arthritis (Tables 9.1 and 9.2).

Early roentgenographic findings in traumatic arthritis are minimal narrowing of the joint space and minimal spur formation superiorly and inferiorly at the junction of the head and neck (Fig. 5.27*A–C*). In later stages the findings are similar to those described for late stages of avascular necrosis (Figs. 3.5*A–C*; 3.10*A–D*; 3.11*A–C*).

Table 9.1
Avascular Necrosis of the Femoral Head—Roentgenographic Findings

A. Early stage
  1. Depression of subchondral cortex of the femoral head
  2. Areas of increased and decreased density throughout the femoral head
  3. Normal cartilaginous joint space
B. Later stage
  1. A defect in the femoral head with irregularity and collapse
  2. Normal cartilaginous joint space
  3. Areas of increased and decreased density throughout the femoral head
C. Advanced stage (may be difficult to differentiate from severe changes of traumatic arthritis)
  1. Marked narrowing of the joint space
  2. Moderate to severe spur formation superiorly and inferiorly
  3. Subchondral cystic formation
  4. Collapse of the femoral head
  5. Acetabular sclerosis

Table 9.2
Traumatic Arthritis of the Hip Joint—Roentgenographic Findings

A. Early stage
  1. Minimal narrowing of the cartilaginous hip space
  2. Minimal spur formation superiorly and anteriorly at the junction of the head and neck
B. Later stage
  1. Advanced narrowing of the cartilaginous joint space
  2. Moderate to severe spur formation
  3. Deformities of the femoral head with subchondral cyst formation
  4. Acetabular sclerosis

Some of the unsatisfactory results among the patients with traumatic arthritis might have been ascribed to avascular necrosis if a more accurate roentgenographic diagnosis had been made. There are cases in which the symptoms and the clinical and roentgenographic findings are more readily explained by joint reactions to trauma (Fig. 9.1A–D).

Findings. There had been an extensive fracture of the acetabulum in which the acetabular walls were severely disrupted, producing a subluxation of the hip joint and far advanced degenerative and proliferative changes in the joint. Degenerative changes were seen as softening of the articular cartilage and a wearing away in a zone about ¾ inches wide that extended over the head of the femur. This zone was ground down and glistening for this reason. With the fracture subluxation most of the stresses between the head of the femur and the acetabulum were taken on the femoral head in this narrow zone. Other portions of the articular surface apparently did not take part in the transference of weight from the head of the femur to the acetabulum. There was a granulation tissue pannus over a considerable portion of the cartilage of the head and this was growing in principally from the periphery at the junction of the cartilage and synovia. The capsule of the joint was extensively thickened and hyperemic.

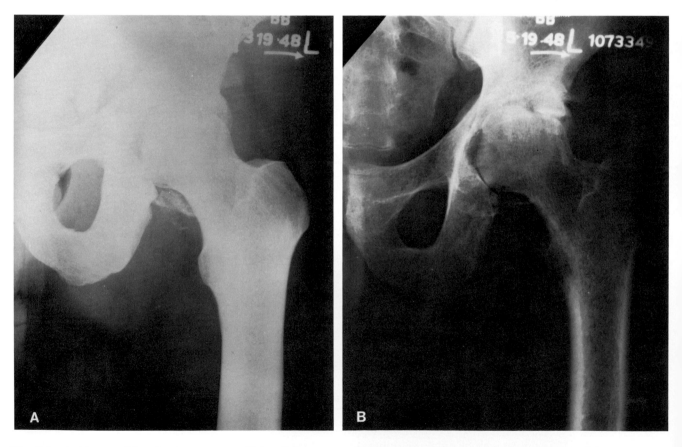

Fig. 9.1   A 38-year-old male in an auto collision February 28, 1948, sustained a severely crushed chest with paradoxical breathing. He was first treated at a private hospital and transferred to LAC-USC Medical Center on March 11, 1948. Three weeks after injury, patient complained of pain in the left hip. Roentgenograms revealed a subluxation of the left hip with marked comminution of the acetabular fragment. A, subluxation of the left hip; roentgenogram taken approximately 3 weeks after his accident. B, roentgenogram 2 months after injury. There is generalized osteoporosis of the head and neck with marked narrowing of the joint space, with fragmentation of the articular surface on the head and acetabulum.

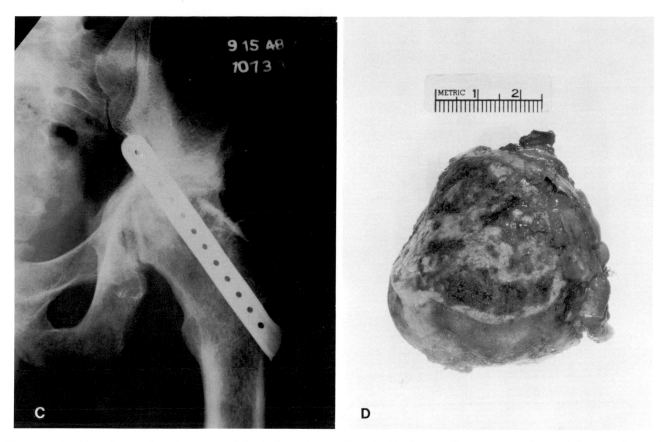

Fig. 9.1 *C,* although an arthroplasty was advised, the patient preferred a hip fusion. *D,* at surgery, advanced degenerative and proliferative changes were observed in the joint. Note the destruction of the cartilage as well as the pannus formation.

Thus, with traumatic synovitis there would be synovial hyperemia and hyperplasia. Destruction of cartilage would take place as a result of subchondral and synovial proliferation and pannus formation. Attrition through motion of the joint would be augmented by incongruity of the joint surfaces or by loose pieces of bone. The hypertrophic underlying bone would give a sclerotic appearance in the roentgenograms. Continuing irritation results in marginal chondro-osseous production with formation of bony spurs and lips. It seems hardly justifiable to attribute all the changes observed in the follow-up roentgenograms solely to avascular necrosis or traumatic arthritis.

In the entire group (Table 9.3) of 531 dislocations with adequate follow-up in this series, including anterior, type I, and fracture-dislocations in adults and children, there were 263 fair or poor results. Eighty-four (16%) had avascular necrosis, 109 (21%) had traumatic arthritis, and 13 (2%) had myositis ossificans of moderate to severe degree.

Of the 13 cases of myositis ossificans three followed simple type I dislocations and two occurred in anterior dislocations (Fig. 3.3), all treated by closed method. Neither early weight-bearing nor immediate active exercises appeared to be a factor in causation of this condition. It appears that hematoma and muscle trauma are factors. Among the eight fracture-dislocations with myositis ossificans, the one type II dislocation was unstable after closed reduction and was opened 8 days later. At surgery, the capsule was shredded and there was considerable hemorrhage in the area (Fig. 3.19*A, B*). Two type III dislocations were opened 21 and 30 days, respectively, after injury. In four type IV dislocations, one was not

Table 9.3
Roentgenographic Joint Changes in 263 Fair or Poor Results According to Type

Type	Total	Fair, clinical x-ray normal	Traumatic arthritis	Avascular necrosis	Myositis ossificans	Infection	Never reduced	Not recognized	Redislocated	Miscellaneous
Anterior	16	1	9	2	2	0	0	0	1	1[a]
Children	9	0	4	4	0	0	0	1[b]	0	0
Type I	47	4	17	20	3	0	2	0	0	1[c]
Type II	23	0	12	6	1	0	1	0	3	0
Type III	82	5	34	21	2	7	4	2	6	1[d]
Type IV	53	0	22	20	4	2	2	2	1	0
Type V	33	2	11	11	1	3	1	2	0	2[e]
Total	263	12	109	84	13	12	10	7	11	5
Percentage			21%	16%	2%					

[a] One neck of femur fractured in attempt at reduction.
[b] One type IV child not recognized with ipsilateral fracture of femur.
[c] One type I irreducible signed out; died in surgery 3 months later.
[d] One type III died in surgery.
[e] Two type V neck of femur fractured in attempt at closed reduction.

Table 9.4
Roentgenographic Joint Changes in 190 Fair or Poor Results (Types II, III, IV, V): Closed, Closed-Opened, Primary Open Reductions

Type	Total	Fair, clinical x-ray normal	Traumatic arthritis	Avascular necrosis	Myositis ossificans	Infections	Never reduced	Not recognized	Redislocations	Miscellaneous
II	22		12	6			1		3	
III	82	5	34	21	2	7	5[a]	2	6	
IV	53	0	22	20	4	2	2	2	1	
V	33	2	11	11	1	3	1[b]	2	0	2[c]
Total	190	7	79	58	7	12	9	6	10	2
Percentage		3%	30%	22%	3%	5%	3%	2%	4%	2%

[a] Neck of femur fractured at closed reduction prior to primary open.
[b] Neck of femur fractured during closed recution
[c] One patient died in surgery during primary open reduction

Table 9.5
Roentgenographic Changes in 33 Fair or Poor Results with Primary Open Reductions

Type	Total	Fair, clinical x-ray normal	Traumatic arthritis	Avascular necrosis	Myositis ossificans	Infections	Never reduced	Not recognized	Redislocated	Miscellaneous
II	1	0	1	0	0	0	0	0	0	0
III	14	1	6	1	1	3	0	0	0	1[a]
IV	9	1	3	3	1	1	0	0	0	0
V	9	0	4	3	0	2	0	0	0	0
Total	22	2	14	7	2	6	0	0	1	1
Percentage			17%	8%		7%				

[a] Patient died in surgery during primary open reduction.

recognized for 2 days and then had a closed reduction. The remaining three patients had primary open reductions, but one patient kept removing the traction because of confusion (Fig. 3.37A–C). In the type V dislocations a closed reduction was accomplished after many attempts, and 4 days later an open procedure was done (Fig. 3.30A–C).

In 57 (11%) of the fair or poor results there were other reasons for the unsatisfactory ratings. There were 12 infections following open procedures (5%). Ten dislocations were never reduced, seven went unrecognized, 11 redislocated after reduction, and five fall into the miscellaneous group. This latter group includes one anterior and two type V cases with the neck of the femur fractured during attempt at closed reduction, one type III patient who died during surgery, one type I with irreducible dislocation who signed out and died 3 months later in an attempt at reconstructive surgery, and a type IV in a child whose hip dislocation was not recognized because of an ipsilateral fracture of the femur.

Twelve cases were rated fair clinically with normal roentgenograms. Clinically, a large majority of patients with fair or poor results have early warning symptoms in less than a year; 60% with avascular necrosis had a painful hip by 1 year, and 40% were painful within 6 months after injury. Of patients with traumatic arthritis, 44% had warning symptoms by the end of the 1st year.

If one were to eliminate the anterior and type I dislocations from this study, the results would be 58 (22%) with avascular necrosis and 79 (30%) with traumatic arthritis in the group of fracture-dislocations (Table 9.4).

The percentage of avascular necrosis in the primary open reductions dropped to 8% and that of traumatic arthritis to 17% (Table 9.5).

These statistics which were analyzed and are statistically significant ($P > 0.05$) are further proof that primary open reductions decreased some of the factors that contribute to avascular necrosis or traumatic arthritis. Removal of bone fragments and debris from the hip joint certainly removes one of the prime factors that may cause traumatic arthritis, namely, an incongruous hip joint.

When operating on a dislocated hip previously reduced by the closed method, one would have to redislocate the hip to adequately visualize the entire hip joint in an effort to properly ascertain the presence or absence of bony fragments, cartilage, or debris. This adds further trauma to an already traumatized hip. I feel that all fracture-dislocations, and also irreducible type I dislocations and those dislocations revealing a wide joint space after reduction of a type I injury, should be opened. Of 176 fracture-dislocations opened, 91% revealed bone fragments, cartilage, and debris in the hip joint, many of the fragments not visualized on the roentgenogram. Tomograms or computerized tomography may be useful in selected cases.[53, 64] More will be discussed on wide joint space after reduction of dislocations in Chapter 10, Prognosis.

Complaints of minor aches and pains should not be ignored. One should appreciate the significance of reflex spasm protecting the hip joint motion at the extremes. A thorough examination is indicated, especially motions of the hip and measurement of the circumference of the thigh. Since a roentgenogram rating is, as a rule, higher than a clinical rating, more weight should be given to apparently minor pathological roentgenographic findings.

Only four patients in this series had ratings of good at 2, 4, 5, and 9 years after injury that required a change in classification to one fair and three poor, 10, 12, 13, and 17 years later because traumatic arthritis developed. Ten patients, after long-term follow-up of more than 10 years, are showing early signs of traumatic arthritis, such as minimal narrowing of the hip joint and spur formation at the junction of the head and neck.

CHAPTER
10

PROGNOSIS

It did not take the author too long to establish as fact that dislocations of the hip, even the simple ones without fractures, are serious injuries. Interest in this hip problem started during the residency years at the University of Southern California Medical Center and has continued since.

There are many factors that determine the prognosis in traumatic dislocations of the hip.

In all dislocations the results are better with early recognition and reduction. Unrecognized dislocations invariably have unsatisfactory results, as do closed reductions attempted more than 72 hours after injury. The prognosis should be guarded when many attempts at closed reduction are done. A widened joint space after a closed reduction in any type of reduction gives a guarded prognosis if immediate arthrotomy is not performed. Loose bodies within the hip joint leaves an incongruous joint space and this leads to traumatic arthritis. Other causes of a widened joint space may be due to soft tissue intervention or to a detached acetabular labrum, and if no arthrotomy is performed the prognosis is definitely guarded.

In type I dislocations, both in children and adults, an insignificant chip fracture about the acetabulum may lead to a guarded prognosis because fragments not visible by roentgenograms may be dislodged from the acetabulum or the femoral head and left in the hip joint. Also, in simple type I dislocations with fractures of the pelvis the results are usually unsatisfactory.

In anterior dislocations with compressions of the femoral head, unsatisfactory results were the rule except for the one anterior type in which a primary open procedure was performed to remove the head fragment (not involving the weight-bearing portion).

Should traumatic dislocations in people over the age of 65 years have a guarded prognosis? There were 19 patients in this age group (with sufficient follow-up). Sixteen had poor results and in three the ratings were good. However, many factors enter into the prognosis. In two patients the neck of the femur was fractured in an attempt at closed reduction, one anterior and the other a type V. One hip dislocation was missed; three hips were left dislocated; one subluxated after a closed reduction; one became infected following an open procedure and an anterior approach was made in a posterior dislocation. Traumatic arthritis or avascular necrosis were responsible for the other unsatisfactory results.

In the 1951 series reported by Thompson and me,[100] there were only 25 open reductions performed with three good results, all in type III dislocations. At that time there was little to be found in the literature concerning early open reduction of fracture-dislocations.

In April 1953, I operated on a patient with a comminuted fracture of the acetabulum associated with dislocation of the hip. Open reduction could not be done until 13 days after injury. At operation many small fragments were removed from the joint and a large fragment of the acetabulum, including the posterior rim, was reduced and held in position by two screws. Twelve months later the result was rated *good* without any evidence of avascular necrosis or traumatic arthritis. The result was still good after a long follow-up.

The favorable result in this case prompted a reevaluation of the previously reported fracture-dislocations. This reevaluation emphasized that poor results occurred when open reduction was delayed or when fracture-dislocations that were presumed to have small, loose fragments within the joint space were treated by closed methods.

The prognoses in the types II, III, IV, and V fracture-dislocations depend upon the type of treatment. In the type II injuries, closed reduction resulted in good results in only 32%; in type III, the incidence of good results was 2%; in type IV, 13%; and in type V there were no good results. The incidence of overall good results in all four types of fracture-dislocations was only 12%.

The prognosis for the fracture-dislocations treated by closed followed by open procedures was better than for those treated by closed reductions. In type II, 54% had good results; in type III, there were, now, 45% with good results; in type IV the results had increased to 31% good; in type V the good results were, now, 33%. The overall percentage of good results had jumped from 12% to 41%.

The prognosis in the fracture-dislocations treated by primary open reduction is much better in types II, III, and V; however, in type IV there is not too much difference in the percentage of good results in those treated by closed followed by open procedures. In type II, although the series is small, there is an 87% incidence of good results.

In type III the good results increased to 67%, and in type V, to 47%. The type IV hips showed only a slight increase in good results, from 31% treated by closed followed by open reduction, to 40% treated by primary open procedures.

In none of the fracture-dislocations were any results rated as excellent. The overall percentage of good results in treatment of all fracture-dislocations by primary open reduction was 60%.

Anterior approaches made for posterior dislocations gave no good results.

CHAPTER
11

NERVE INJURIES

Sixty-eight nerve injuries were encountered in this series (Table 11.1); that is in approximately 8% of the 830 dislocations of the hip. There were no nerve injuries in the anterior dislocations. The sciatic paralysis previously reported occurring in an anterior dislocation was in error.

Three sciatic injuries in children (two, type IV; one, type I) returned to normal within 1 year.

There were 18 nerve injuries in type I dislocations in adults—8 sciatic and 10 peroneal. Two patients still had nerve dysfunction 7 months later; in one patient nerve dysfunction was still present at 39 months and one patient had persistent palsy 6 years after his injury. Six patients returned to normal within 3 to 12 months. Eight cases were lost to follow-up.

Forty-seven (13%) of the 68 nerve injuries were encountered in 368 fracture-dislocations of the hip (Table 11.2). The sciatic nerve was involved in 16 cases and the peroneal nerve in 31. Open reductions were performed for 31 of the 47 dislocations with nerve injuries. The findings in these 31 cases were as follows: There was definite contusion of the nerve in 11 (nine type III, and two type IV. There was a partial nerve laceration in two; one was a type IV and the other a type III). In another patient with a type V lesion the femoral head was pressing on the sciatic nerve but the nerve appeared to be normal. In three others, there was no gross evidence of nerve damage, but at operation the sciatic nerve was lying over a bone fragment. In two of the 31 patients with sciatic paralysis and posterior fracture-dislocations, anterior approaches were made without any attempt to visualize the nerve. In the remaining 12 cases of nerve injury the operative note made no mention of the sciatic nerve in four, and in eight stated that the nerve was identified and retracted during surgery, but did not mention whether the nerve was traumatized.

Six patients with type III lesions had no sciatic or peroneal palsy but showed evidence of trauma to the nerve at the time of surgery. In one the sciatic nerve was stretched over the femoral head; in another the nerve was thinned out over the top of the femoral head; in the third the nerve was dissected free of callus 21 days after surgery; in the fourth there was hemorrhage around the nerve with a displaced bone fragment pressing against it; and in the other two the sciatic nerve was contused.

One patient with type III nerve injury had exploration of the sciatic nerve 9 months after a closed reduction of the dislocation, with return of function 9

Table 11.1
Distribution of Associated Nerve Injuries in 830 Traumatic Dislocations of the Hip

Dislocation		Nerve injuries					
Type	Number	Sciatic	Peroneal	Total	Returned to normal	Did not return to normal	Insurricient follow-up
Anterior	93	0	0	0	0	0	0
Children	75	3	0	3	3	0	0
Type I	276	8	10	18	6	4	8
Type II	62	3	4	7	3	2	2
Type III	174	8	14	22	11	7	4
Type IV	77	4	8	12	4	7	1
Type V	55	1	5	6	2	2	2
Deaths	18	0	0	0	0	0	0
Total	830	27	41	68	29 (43%)	22 (32%)	17 (25%)

months after exploration. At surgery the nerve was surrounded by adhesions which were freed. The blood supply to the nerve appeared normal.

Of the 68 injured nerves, 29 (43%) had returned to normal 2 months to 5 years after injury; 22 (32%) had failed to recover or had recovered partially; and in 17 (25%) the result was unknown because of insufficient follow-up.

Correlation of the type of fracture-dislocation, the nerve involved, and the result revealed the following:

In the 62 type II cases there were three sciatic and four peroneal lesions. One sciatic and one peroneal nerve failed to recover completely and two were unknown because of insufficient follow-up.

In the 224 type III cases there were eight sciatic and 14 peroneal lesions. Function returned to normal in four sciatic and seven peroneal nerve lesions, failed to return to normal in seven (two sciatic and five peroneal), and was not known because of insufficient follow-up in four.

In the 74 type IV cases there were four sciatic and eight peroneal nerve lesions. Function returned to normal in four nerves (one sciatic and three peroneal), failed to return in seven (three sciatic and four peroneal), and was unknown in one because of insufficient follow-up.

In the 55 type V cases there were five peroneal nerve lesions and one sciatic. Function returned to normal in two (one sciatic, one peroneal), failed to return in two, and was unknown in two because of insufficient follow-up.

The most important factor in the production of nerve injury in type I dislocation may be the marked internal rotation of the hip that occurs at the time of dislocation. This rotation causes a winding and tightening of the sciatic nerve. The circumduction method of reducing a dislocated hip may also be a cause of nerve injury. In fracture-dislocations the most probable cause of nerve injury is direct pressure on the sciatic nerve caused by the femoral head or an acetabular fragment.

It is important to examine a patient for sciatic or peroneal palsy prior to reduction of a dislocation. If this condition is found, urgent, timely reduction of the dislocation is indicated.

Table 11.2
Distribution of Associated Nerve Injuries in 368 Fracture-Dislocations of the Hip

Dislocation		Nerve injuries					
Type	Number	Sciatic	Peroneal	Total	Returned to normal[a]	Did not return to normal[b]	Insufficient follow-up[c]
II	62	3	4	7	3	2	2
III	174	8	14	22	11	7	4
IV	77	4	8	12	4	7	1
V	55	1	5	6	2	2	2
Total	368	16	31	47	20	18	9

[a] 43% of nerve injuries returned to normal within 3 to 30 months.
[b] 28% did not return to normal.
[c] 19% were unknown because of insufficient follow-up.

PROCEDURES

Operator: H. C. Epstein, M.D.

Preoperative Diagnosis: Fracture-dislocation, posterior, left hip with sciatic palsy (peroneal portion), nerve intact

Procedure 11.1

The posterior acetabulum was comminuted and fractured into several pieces. Two small pieces, neither of which contained more than ½ cm of articular surface were freed and removed. The larger pieces were in essentially their anatomical position and were left without specific internal fixation. The acetabulum was irrigated, and cartilage in general appeared to be normal. The ligamentum teres was severed and was freed in the acetabulum. The sciatic nerve appeared grossly to be intact. It was adjacent to the femoral head. Through a posterior incision beginning about 2 inches below and lateral to the posterior-superior iliac spine and extending along in the direction of the gluteus maximus muscle to the area of the greater trochanter and then down laterally for 2½ inches, incision was made and carried down to the subcutaneous tissue. Bleeding vessels were clamped and electrocoagulated. Beneath this, the gluteus maximus was divided in the direction of its fibers in the proximal portion of the wound and distally the aponeurosis of the gluteus maximus and the fascia lata was incised in the direction of the skin incision. Immediately below this was the prominent posteriorly dislocated femoral head. In order to manipulate the femoral head and demonstrate the sciatic nerve it was necessary to detach the external rotator muscle. This was done and reflected medially, protecting the sciatic nerve. Also the posterior-superior one-half of the insertion in the gluteus maximus muscle into the greater trochanter was necessarily detached. The acetabulum was visualized and irrigated with saline. It was noted as described above. The hip was reduced manually and gently, until firm on reduction. The remaining fragments in the posterior end of the fracture fell into essentially anatomical position and were held there by firm muscular fixation and left *in situ*. The sciatic nerve demonstrated, again at this point, appeared grossly in continuity without evidence of significant trauma and was left, after it was protected during the procedure. External rotators were repaired with figure-of-8 No. 0 chromic sutures. The posterior portion of the gluteus medius insertion was repaired with interrupted No. 0 chromic sutures. The fascia lata and gluteus maximus muscle were repaired with interrupted running No. 0 chromic sutures. Subcutaneous tissue was closed with No. 3-0 plain catgut suture, and the skin with running No. 32 wire. Estimated blood loss 200 ml. The patient tolerated the procedure well. No blood replacement was needed during the operation. Postoperatively he was stable; he was awake and was placed in Buck's extension and returned to the ward. Both pre- and postoperatively it was explained to the patient that there is perhaps 50% chance of return of peroneal nerve function and that there is a significant chance for aseptic necrosis and/or degenerative arthritis of the femoral head.

Operator: H. C. Epstein, M.D.

Preoperative Diagnosis: Unstable acetabular fracture of the left femur; displaced fragment of posterior acetabular rim was pressing against sciatic nerve with hemorrhage into tissue surrounding nerve; *no sciatic paralysis*

Procedure 11.2

Under general anesthesia the left hip was examined and noted to be unstable, easily dislocating with flexion of the hip. With the hip in the dislocated position the patient was turned to the right lateral decubitus position and the left hip prepared and draped in the usual manner. An Austin Moore incision was made over the posterolateral aspect of the hip and carried through subcutaneous tissue and fascia. The fascia of the gluteus maximus was exposed and with the use of the Mayo scissors was incised along the direction of the skin incision. The gluteus maximus fibers were separated along the line of their course. The subgluteal fat pad was exposed and the sciatic nerve identified. There was noted to be a large amount of hemorrhage into the tissue around the sciatic nerve, with the displaced fragment of the posterior acetabular rim pressing against the sciatic nerve. The incision was extended down through the torn capsule, exposing the femoral head. It was noted that the femoral head on the posteromedial aspect was excoriated considerably. Two small fragments of bone were removed from the acetabulum with their attached pieces of cartilage. A large fracture of the posterior acetabular rim was noted and was comminuted, there being two pieces. The smaller piece was removed and measured approximately 1 × 1 cm. The larger piece was approximately 6 × 3 cm in a triangular pattern. The acetabulum was irrigated and loose clots and fibrous tissue were removed. The ligamentum teres was noted to be torn. The soft tissue about the edges of the fracture fragment and the place where it had been torn loose from the acetabulum were dissected free, exposing the edges of fracture. The fracture piece was replaced in anatomical position and held there with two 2-inch screws directed posteromedially. The wound was then irrigated. Next, the capsule of the joint was reduced after the hip was relocated and after it was repaired with No. 0 chromic interrupted suture. X-rays taken at surgery revealed that the screws were definitely not in the acetabulum but were transfixing the fractured fragment and holding it in good position. The rotators were then approximated to their attachment at the greater trochanter with interrupted No. 0 chromic suture. The fascia over the gluteus maximus was approximated with interrupted No. 0 chromic suture. The subcutaneous tissue was approximated with No. 000 plain interrupted suture and the skin was closed with No. 000 nylon interrupted suture. Estimated blood loss was 400 ml; no blood was given. The patient tolerated the procedure well and left the operating room in satisfactory condition. X-rays taken prior to waking the patient revealed that the two screws were in excellent position and that the hip was well reduced. The patient was transferred to a traction bed while at surgery.

Operator: H. C. Epstein, M.D.

Preoperative Diagnosis: Posterior fracture-dislocation of left acetabulum; complete paralysis of sciatic nerve secondary to hip dislocation; complete sciatic paralysis, nerve intact

Procedure 11.3

Open reduction and internal fixation of fracture-dislocation of left hip: under satisfactory general anesthesia, with patient in prone position, a Gibson approach was made through deep fascia along the upper border of the gluteus maximus. The short external rotators were cut at their insertion to afford better exposure of the hip joint. One small fragment of bone was found in the acetabulum and was removed. The only other fragment, comprising virtually all of the posterior and superior aspects of the acetabululm and including the triangular articular surface, measured about 3 cm on a side. After thorough irrigation of the joint, the femoral head was reduced and the fragment replaced anatomically and fixed by two screws at approximately right angles to each other. The articular surface of the femoral head showed two faint lines across the cartilage but no actual loss of cartilage or apparent fracture. The sciatic nerve emerging from the sciatic notch was found to lie across the corner of the fragment, but careful inspection of the nerve did not reveal hematoma within the nerve or laceration of its fibers or sheath. Palpation of the nerve did not identify edema or defect. Internal rotation tended to move the acetabular fragment some and it was determined to hold the extremity in external rotation postoperatively. Short rotators were reattached at their insertion by interrupted No. 0 chromic pulley sutures. One loose chromic pulley suture was used to reapproximate the divided 1-inch-wide border of the gluteus medius which had apparently been cut by the displaced acetabular fragment. Deep fascia and fascia lata were closed with interrupted No. 00 chromic sutures, skin with No. 25 stainless steel wire. Streptomycin (1 gm) and 1,000,000 units of penicillin were injected into the vicinity of the acetabulum. During the procedure, care was taken not to put undue pressure or traction on the injured sciatic nerve; care was also taken not to remove any of the soft tissue attachments to the acetabular fragment. Procedure was well tolerated by the patient and he was returned to ward in good condition.

Operator: H. C. Epstein, M.D.

Preoperative Diagnosis: Fracture-dislocation of the left hip, type III; Transverse fracture, left femur; transverse fracture, left humerus; fracture of clavicle; multiple fractured ribs; complete sciatic palsy, nerve appeared normal

Procedure 11.4

Under adequate general anesthesia, with the patient in the lateral position on his right side, a midlateral incision was made over the thigh to expose the fracture site. This was done by following the lateral intermuscular septum down to bone. The integrity of the vastus lateralis was not violated during this dissection. The fracture site was found and the hematoma cleaned out. A Hansen Street nail was then inserted retrograde into the proximal fragment, brought out through a second incision over the buttock, and then driven into the distal fragment. However, the diameter of this nail was found to be too small so it was withdrawn and two nested Küntscher nails (11 mm × 42 cm) were inserted. The fracture had been anatomically reduced and there was good stability, both rotatory and angulatory, at the fracture site after the nails had been driven home. The wound was closed in the routine manner with No. 00 chromic to the fascia and No. 35 wire to the skin. Dry sterile pressure dressing was applied and the patient was then turned into the prone position. The left buttock was then prepared and after regowning and regloving, an open reduction of the hip was undertaken through an oblique incision extending from the posterosuperior iliac spine to the greater trochanter. The gluteus maximus was split by blunt dissection. The sciatic nerve was then isolated. *Preoperatively complete (motor and sensory) peroneal palsy and complete motor sciatic palsy were present.* The sciatic nerve was easily found and retracted by means of umbilical tape. Two No. 1 silk ligatures were placed in the tendon of the piriformis and the tendon was cut between the ligatures. The remainder of the short rotator muscles were detached from the greater trochanter. At this point considerable difficulty was encountered in cleaning out the acetabulum. Because of the fact that the femoral neck and head lay directly over the acetabulum, it was only with difficulty that the acetabulum itself could be digitally explored and cleaned out. During the process, traction had to be placed on the femur and a loud cracking noise was heard. X-rays subsequently showed that this was due to fracture of the femur near the previous fracture site and resulted in a rather large butterfly fragment, the position of which, however, was virtually anatomical. Nonetheless, the operator was finally able to satisfy himself that the contents of the acetabulum had been cleaned out. The femoral head was then reduced. A large oblique fracture of the posterior rim of the acetabulum was present; however, the major portion of this fragment was composed of articular cartilage. There was not enough bone present in the fragment to enable it to be replaced and held with a screw, therefore it was sutured into position with No. 1 chromic catgut. The wound was irrigated with 1,000,000 units of penicillin and 1 g of streptomycin in 100 ml of saline. The wound was closed in layers after the tendon of the piriformis had been reattached. Dry sterile dressing was applied, and the patient left surgery in good condition.

CHAPTER
12

RECONSTRUCTIVE HIP OPERATIONS

Hip surgery, other than open reduction, was performed on 25 patients. None was performed as a primary procedure. The procedures and results are tabulated in Table 12.1

Arthrodesis, successful in 11 of the 12 cases, was usually advised because it offered greater assurance of a painless, stable hip. This is in agreement with Phemister,[83] who stated that arthrodesis is the procedure of choice and that the extensive stripping of the capsule, entailed by the procedure for cup arthroplasty, led to the poor results.

Two of the patients with good results following cup arthroplasties have had follow-up of less than 2 years. One of the poor results subluxated after operation, but the patient refused further treatment. Two patients became infected and the cup was subsequently removed. The other two patients with cup arthroplasties have had persistent hip pain.

Harris[45] concluded that mold arthroplasty is the treatment of choice for most patients who require operation for traumatic arthritis following traumatic dislocation of hips. Brav,[9] in his series, included five cup arthroplasties (two primary) with good results in four, and five arthrodeses with good results in three cases.

Although the method of arthrodesis was more successful in this group, the series was too small to permit significant comparison of the merits of arthroplasty and arthrodesis.

Three arthrodeses were performed at 1, 3, and 4 months after injury. The remaining patients were arthrodesed many months later because of disability after traumatic arthritis or aseptic necrosis.

Two cup arthroplasties were performed for unrecognized dislocations 3 and 6 months after injury, both with unsatisfactory results.

In addition to the 25 reconstructive procedures previously discussed, seven total hip implants have been done during the past 4 years, with good results in six patients and insufficient follow-up in one 23-year-old man who had a Wagner procedure following a missed dislocation 8 months after injury. One patient was a woman 40 years of age; the rest were over 60 years of age. There were no primary total hip implants. Two procedures, a type IV and a type V, were performed more than 18 years after the first injury; one followed a successful cup

Table 12.1
Reconstructive Hip Operations

Procedure	Type of dislocation	Results			Average length of follow-up (months)
		Good	Poor	Total	
Cup arthroplasty	I	1	0	1	12
	III	2	3	5	90
	IV	0	2	2	114
Hip fusion	I	4	0	4	78
	III	1	1	2	12
	IV	2	0	2	162
	V	4	0	4	30
Fascial arthroplasty	V	0	1	0	12
Austin Moore prosthesis	V	1	0	1	7
Judet prosthesis	V	1	2	3	78
Totals		16	9	25	51

arthroplasty of 12 years because of severe hip pain (type III), and the other (also a type III) was performed after a cup arthroplasty of 7 years' duration because of severe hip pain. The other two implants were done approximately 2 years after injury in a type I because of avascular necrosis and because of severe traumatic arthritis in a type IV dislocation.

Primary arthrodesis, cup arthroplasty, or total hip implant is rarely indicated. Many patients with traumatic arthritis or avascular necrosis were satisfied with their results even though there was some hip discomfort. Seven patients with moderate to severe pain and disability were recommended for secondary procedures but refused further operations. It may be, however, that relief was obtained at other institutions.

CHAPTER
13

SUMMARY

This monograph is based on a study of 830 traumatic dislocated hips, both anterior and posterior, in adults and children.

All traumatic dislocations of the hip must be treated as an emergency. Recognition and reduction in under 24 hours gives a better prognosis. Therefore, routine roentgenograms of the pelvis must be taken in all accident cases with major injuries in order to avoid overlooking a dislocation. The majority of traumatic dislocations of the hip are usually the result of a motor vehicle accident in which multiple trauma engenders a life-threatening situation which diverts attention from the hip. Coma, fracture of the ipsilateral femur or tibia, or dislocation or fracture of the contralateral hip may obscure important clinical diagnostic clues.

Multiple attempts at closed reduction are contraindicated in both anterior and posterior dislocations. Closed reduction of simple type I injuries performed 72 hours or longer after injury all led to poor results.

The majority of patients with type I posterior and simple anterior dislocations walked by the 2nd month. There was no evidence that early weight-bearing increased the percentage of avascular necrosis or traumatic arthritis.

The prognosis in type I injuries with fractures of the pelvis and in those chip fractures off the posterior acetabulum should be guarded. In the latter cases small fragments not visible by roentgenograms may be dislodged from the acetabulum or the femoral head and dislodged into the hip joint with a resultant traumatic arthritis. Roentgenograms should be taken of the pelvis after all closed reductions to check for concentric reductions. Any widening of the joint space should alert the orthopaedist to loose fragments or soft tissue intervention such as a detached acetabular labrium or a buttonholing of the femoral head through the capsule, or, as recently reported, to a piriformis muscle displaced across the acetabulum. Any widening of the joint space demands an immediate arthrotomy.

The results in posterior type I dislocations in adults were 65% excellent-good, and 35% fair or poor. Avascular necrosis occurred in 15% and traumatic arthritis in 13%.

The results in the anterior dislocations were 70% excellent-good and 30% fair or poor. Avascular necrosis occurred in 4% and traumatic arthritis in 17%, with the majority of the latter occurring in the dislocations with compressions of the femoral head.

In children's dislocations all anterior types were excellent-good. In the posterior type I group, four had fair results, the rest being excellent or good. Avascular necrosis occurred in one type I and in two fracture-dislocations (6%). Traumatic arthritis was evident in six cases, three in simple dislocations and three in fracture-dislocations (12%). Fracture-dislocations in children should be treated in the same manner as for the adult, i.e., primary open reduction.

In the types II, III, IV, and V fracture-dislocations, primary open reductions appeared to give better results than did closed reduction, or closed reduction followed by open procedures. The objective of primary open reduction is to remove loose fragments and stabilize an unstable hip joint. By doing the above procedure the appearance of traumatic arthritis is delayed and its severity minimized. In the overall treatment of traumatic dislocations, the incidence of avascular necrosis was 21%; in traumatic arthritis, 16%. In the group of fracture-dislocations, avascular necrosis was evident in 22% and traumatic arthritis in 30%.

When primary open reductions were performed on these fracture-dislocations, the percentage of avascular necrosis dropped to 8% and that of traumatic arthritis fell to 17%.

Anterior approaches for open reduction of posterior dislocations are contraindicated.

Primary arthrodesis or cup arthroplasty is rarely indicated. Many patients with traumatic arthritis or avascular necrosis were satisfied with their results even though there was some hip discomfort. However, total hip replacement is probably the reconstructive procedure of choice.

Of the 68 nerve injuries, 29 (43%) had returned to normal 2 months to 5 years after injury; 22 (32%) had failed to recover or had recovered partially; and in 17 (25%) the result was unknown because of insufficient follow-up. Prompt reduction in a simple type I dislocation and primary open reduction in a fracture-dislocation are indicated in patients with sciatic or peroneal palsy.

Since the majority of dislocations in this series were due to automobile accidents the use of seatbelts could have prevented many of these serious injuries.

BIBLIOGRAPHY

1. Aggarwal, N. D., and Singh, H. Unreduced anterior dislocation of the hip; report of seven cases. *J Bone Joint Surg (Br)* 49: 288–92, 1967.
2. Allis, O. H. *Difficulties Encountered in the Reduction of Dislocation of the Hip*, pp. 164–167. Dornan, Philadelphia, 1896.
3. Armstrong, J. R. Traumatic dislocation of the hip joint. J Bone Joint Surg 30: 430–445, 1948.
4. Aufranc, O. E., Jones, W. N., and Harris, W. Recurrent traumatic dislocation of the hip in a child. *JAMA 190 (4):* 291–294, 1964.
5. Aufranc, O. E., Jones, W. S., Turner, R. H., and Thomas, W. H. Fracture of the acetabulum with dislocation of the hip and sciatic palsy; fracture of the month. *JAMA 201 (4):* 690–691, 1967.
6. Banks, S. W. Aseptic necrosis of the femoral head following traumatic dislocation of the hip. *J. Bone Joint Surg 23:* 753–781, 1941.
7. Bernhang, A. M. Simultaneous bilateral traumatic dislocation of the hip in a child. *J. Bone Joint Surg (Am) 52 (2):* 365–366, 1970.
8. Brighton, C. T. Personal communication.
9. Brav, E. A. Traumatic dislocation of the hip; Army experience and results over a twelve year period. *J. Bone Joint Surg 44:* 1115–1134, 1962.
10. Buchanan, J. J. Open reduction of old dislocation of the hip. *Surg Gynecol Obstet 31:* 462–471, 1920.
11. Byram, G., *et al.* Traumatic dislocation of the hip in children. *South Med J 60:* 805–10, 1967.
12. Campbell, W. C. Posterior dislocation of the hip with fracture of the acetabulum. *J Bone Joint Surg 18:* 842–850, 1936.
12a. Canale, S. T., and Manugian, A. H. *Irreducible traumatic dislocations, J Bone Joint Surg (Am) 61:* 11, 7–14, 1979.
13. Choyce, C. C. Traumatic dislocation of the hip in childhood and relation of trauma to pseudocoxalgia. *Br J Surg 12:* 52–59, 1924.
14. Clarke, H. O. Traumatic dislocation of the hip joint in a child. *Br J Surg 16:* 690–692, 1929.
15. Dameron, T. B. Bucket-handle tear of acetabular labrum accompanying posterior dislocation of the hip. *J Bone Joint Surg (Am) 41:* 1, 1959.
16. Dehne, E., and Immerman, E. W. Dislocation of the hip combined with fracture of the shaft of the femur on the same side. *J Bone Joint Surg (Am) 33:* 731–745, 1951.
17. Dencker, H. Traumatic dislocation of the hip with fracture of the shaft of the ipsilateral femur. *Acta Chir Scand 129:* 593–596, 1965.
18. Dingley, D. Pubic dislocation of the hip. *J Bone Joint Surg (Am) 46:* 865, 1964.
19. Dollinger, J. The reposition of inverterbrate traumatic luxation of the hip joint. *Ann Surg 55:* 176–180, 1912.
20. Duncan, C. P., and Shim, S. S. Blood supply of the head of the femur in traumatic hip dislocation. *Surg Gynecol Obstet 144:* 185–191, 1977.
21. Eichenholtz, S. N., and Stark, R. M. Central acetabular fractures; a review of thirty-five cases. *J Bone and Joint Surg (Am) 46:* 695, 1964.
22. Elliott, R. B. Central fractures of the acetabulum. *Clin Orthop 7:* 189–201, 1956.
23. Epstein, H. C. Traumatic dislocation of the hip. *Clin Orthop 92:* 116–142, 1973.
24. Epstein, H. C. Traumatic anterior and simple posterior dislocations of the hip in adults and children. A.A.O.S. Instructional Course Lectures, vol. 22, pp 115–145. Mosby, St. Louis, 1973.
25. Epstein, H. C. Posterior fracture-dislocation of the hip. *J Bone Joint Surg (Am) 56:* 1103–1127, 1974.
26. Epstein, H. C. Posterior fracture-dislocations of the hip; comparison of open and closed methods of treatment in certain types. *J Bone Joint Surg (Am) 43:* 1079–1098, 1961.
27. Epstein, H. C. (Discussor with Harris, W. H., Jones W. N., and Aufranc, O. E. Fracture of the month: fracture-dislocation of the hip), Grand Rounds at Massachusetts General Hospital. *JAMA 186:* 1160–1163, 1963.
28. Epstein, H. C. Posterior fracture-dislocations of the hip. *J Bone Joint Surg (Am), 56:* 6, 1974.
29. Epstein, H. C., and Harvey, J. P. Anterior dislocations of the hip. *Orthop Rev. 1:* 1, 1972.
29a. Ferguson, A. B., and Howarth, M. D.: Coxa magna. *JAMA 104:* 808–812, 1935.
30. Freeman, G. E., Jr. Traumatic dislocation of the hip in children; a report of seven cases and review of the literature. *J Bone Joint Surg (Am) 43:* 401–406, 1961.
31. Funk, F. J. Traumatic dislocation of the hip in children; factors influencing prognosis and treatment. *J Bone and Joint Surg (Am) 44:* 1135–1145, 1962.
32. Funsten, R. V., Kinser, P., and Frankel, C. J. Dashboard dislocation of the hip; a report of twenty cases of traumatic dislocation. *J Bone Joint Surg 20:* 124–132, 1938.
33. Garden, R. S. Malreduction and avascular necrosis in subcapital fractures of the femur. *J Bone Joint Surg (Br) 53:* 193, 1971.
34. Garrett, J. C., *et al.* Treatment of late, unreduced, traumatic posterior dislocation of the hip. *J Bone Joint Surg (Am) 61:* 2–6, 1979.
35. Ghormley, R. K., and Sullivan, R. Traumatic dislocation of the hip. *Am. J Surg 85:* 298–305, 1953.
36. Glass, A., and Powell, H. D. W. Traumatic dislocation of the hip in children. *J Bone Joint Surg 43:* 29–36, 1961.
37. Glynn, P. Two cases of traumatic dislocation of the hip in children. *Lancet 1:* 1093–1094, 1932.
38. Gordon, E. J., and Freiberg, J. A. Posterior dislocation of the hip with fracture of the head of the femur. *J Bone Joint Surg (Am) 31:* 869–872, 1949.
39. Griswold, R. A., and Herd, C. R. Dislocation of hip with fracture of posterior rim of acetabulum. *J Indiana State Med Assoc 22:* 150–153, 1929.
40. Haines, C. Traumatic dislocation of head of femur in a child. *J Bone Joint Surg 10:* 1126–1127, 1937.
41. Haliburton, R. A., Brockenshire, F. A., and Barber, J. R. Avascular necrosis of the femoral capital epiphysis after traumatic dislocation of the hip in children. *J Bone Joint Surg (BR), 43:* 43–46, 1961.

42. Hamada, G. Unreduced anterior dislocation of the hip. *J Bone Joint Surg (Br) 39:* 471–476, 1957.

43. Hammond, G. Posterior dislocation of hip associated with fracture. *Proc R Soc Med 37:* 281, 1944.

44. Hampson, W. F. J. Venous obstruction by anterior dislocation of the hip joint. *Br J Accident Surg 4 (1):* 69–73, 1972.

45. Harris, W. H. Traumatic arthritis of the hip after dislocation and acetabular fractures; treatment by mold arthroplasty. *J Bone Joint Surg (Am), 51:* 737, 1969.

46. Hart, V. L. Fracture-dislocation of the hip. *J Bone Joint Surg 24 (2):* 458–460, 1942.

47. Haw, D. W. Complications following fracture-dislocation of the hip. *Br Med J 5442:* 1111–1112, 1965.

48. Helal, B., *et al.* Unrecognized dislocation of the hip in fractures of the femoral shaft. *J Bone Joint Surg (Br) 49:* 293–300, 1967.

49. Henderson, R. S. Traumatic anterior dislocation of the hip. *J Bone Joint Surg (Br) 33:* 602–603, 1951.

50. Henry, A. K., and Bayumi, M. Fracture of the femur with luxation of the ipsilateral hip. *Br J Surg 22:* 204, 1934.

51. Howe, W. W., Lacey, T., and Schwartz, R. P. A study of the gross anatomy of the arteries supplying the proximal portion of the femur and the acetabulum. *J Bone Joint Surg (Am) 32:* 856–866, 1950.

52. Huckstep, R. C. Neglected traumatic dislocation of the hip. *J Bone Joint Surg (Br) 53:* 355.

53. Jazayeri, M. Posterior fracture-dislocation of the hip joint with emphasis on the importance of hip tomography in their management. *Orthop. Rev., 7 (3):* 59–64, 1978.

54. Judet, R., Judet, J., LaGrange, J., and Dunoyer, J. A study of the arterial vascularization of the femoral neck in the adult. *J Bone Joint Surg (Am) 37:* 663–680, 1955.

55. Judet, R., Judet, J., and Letournel, E. Fractures of the acetabulum; classification and surgical approaches for open reduction. *J Bone Joint Surg (Am) 46:* 1615–1646, 1964.

56. Katznelson, A. N. Traumatic anterior dislocation of the hip. *J Bone Joint Surg (Br), 44:* 129–130, 1962.

57. Kelly, P. J., and Lipscomb, R. R. Primary vitallium-mold arthroplasty for posterior dislocation of the hip with fracture of the femoral head. *J Bone Joint Surg (Am) 40:* 675, 1958.

58. Kelly, R. P., and Yarbrough, S. H., III. Posterior fracture-dislocation of the femoral head with retained medial head fragment. *J Trauma 11:* 97–108, 1971.

59. Key, J. A., and Conwell, H. E., *Management of Fractures, Dislocations and Sprains*, ed. 7. Mosby, St. Louis, 1961.

60. King, D., and Richards, V. Fracture-dislocation of the hip joint. *J Bone Joint Surg 23:* 327, 1941.

61. Kleiman, S. G., Stevens, J., Kolb, L., and Pankovich, A. Late sciatic nerve palsy following posterior fracture-dislocation of the hip. *J Bone Joint Surg (Am) 53:* 781–782, 1971.

62. Knight, R. A., and Smith, M. Central fractures of the acetabulum. *J Bone Joint Surg (Am) 40:* 1–16, 1958.

63. Lars-Olof, L. Traumatic dislocation of the hip; follow-up on cases from Stockholm area. *Acta Orthop Scand 41:* 188–198, 1970.

64. Lasda, N. A., Levinsohn, E. M., Yuan, H. A., and Burnell, W. P. Computerized tomography in disorders of the hip. *J Bone Joint Surg (Am) 60:* 8, 1978.

65. Lauber, A. Aseptic necrosis of the femoral head. *J Mt Sinai Hosp 24:* 18, 1957.

66. Levine, M. A. A treatment of central fractures of the acetabulum. *J Bone Joint Surg 25:* 902–906, 1943.

67. Litton, L. O., and Workman, C. Traumatic anterior dislocation of the hip in children. *J Bone Joint Surg (Am) 40:* 1419–1422, 1958.

68. Mason, M. L. Traumatic dislocation of the hip in childhood; report of a case. *J Bone Joint Surg (Br) 36:* 630–632, 1954.

69. McFarland, J. A. Anterior dislocation of the hip. *J Surg 23:* 607, 1935.

70. Meyerding, H. W., and Walker, H. R. Fracture-dislocation of the acetabular rim with dislocation of the hip and traumatic sciatic paralysis. *Int Surg 13:* 539, 1950.

71. Miller, C. H. Traumatic hip dislocation, treatment and results. *Minn Med. 54:* 253–260, 1971.

72. Moore, J. R. Old traumatic dislocation of the hip with malunited fracture of the acetabulum. *Surg Clin North Am 33:* 1551, 1953.

73. Moore, T. M., Hill, J. V., and Harvey, J. P. Central acetabular fracture secondary to epileptic seizure. *J Bone Joint Surg (Am) 52:* 7, 1459–1462, 1970.

74. Morton, K. S. Traumatic dislocation of the hip in children. *Br J Surg 47:* 233–237, 1969.

75. Nicoll, E. A. Traumatic dislocation of the hip joint. *J Bone Joint Surg (Br) 34:* 503, 1952.

76. Niloff, P., and Petrie, J. G. Traumatic anterior dislocation of the hip. *Can. Med. Assoc J 62:* 574–576, 1950.

77. Nixon, J. R. Late open reduction of traumatic dislocation of the hip; report of three cases. *J Bone Joint Surg (Br) 58:* 1, 1976.

78. Paus, B. Traumatic dislocation of the hip—late results in 76 cases. *Acta Orthop Scand 21:* 99–112, 1951.

79. Pearson, J. R., and Horgacton, E. J. Fractures of the pelvis involving the floor of the acetabulum, *J Bone Joint Surg (Br) 44:* 550–561, 1962.

80. Pearson, D. E., and Mann, R. J. Traumatic hip dislocation in children. *Clin Orthop 92:* 189–194, 1973.

81. Pennsylvania Orthopaedic Society. Traumatic dislocation of the hip joint in children; a report by the Scientific Research Committee. *J Bone Joint Surg (Am) 42:* 705–710, 1960.

82. Pennsylvania Orthopaedic Society. Traumatic dislocation of the hip joint in children; final report. *J Bone Joint Surg (Am) 50:* 79–88, 1968.

83. Phemister, D. B. Fractures of neck of femur, dislocations of hip and obscure vascular disturbances producing aseptic necrosis of head of femur. *Surg Gynecol Obstet 59:* 415–440, 1934.

84. Piggot, J. Traumatic dislocation of the hip in childhood. *J Bone Joint Surg (Br) 43:* 38–42, 1961.

85. Pipkin, G. Treatment of grade IV fracture-dislocation of the hip; a review. *J Bone Joint Surg (Am) 39:* 1027–1042, 1957.

86. Potts, F. N., and Obletz, B. E. Aseptic necrosis of head of femur following traumatic dislocation. *J Bone Joint Surg 21:* 101–110, 1939.

87. Powers, J. A., and Bach, P. J. Coxa magna. *South Med J 70:* 1297–1299, 1977.

88. Raine, G. E. T. Acute traumatic dislocation of a con-

genital dysplastic hip; case report. *J Bone Joint Surg (Br)* 55: 640, 1973.

89. Rowe, C. R., and Lowell, J. D. Prognosis of fractures of the acetabulum. *J Bone Joint Surg (Am)* 43: 30, 1961.

90. Scham, S. M., *et al.* Traumatic anterior dislocation of the hip with fracture of the femoral head; a case report. *Clin Orthop* 62: 133–135, 1969.

91. Schlonsky, J., and Miller, P. R. Traumatic dislocation of hip in children. *J Bone Joint Surg (Am)* 55: 1057–1063

92. Scott, J. E., and Thomas F. B. Delayed presentation of post-traumatic posterior dislocation of the hip with acetabular rim fracture. *Injury* 5: 325–326, 1974.

93. Siffert, R. S. Personal communication.

93a. Sledge, C. B. Personal communication.

94. Speed, Kellog: Simultaneous bilateral traumatic dislocation of the hip. *Am J Surg* 85: 292–297, 1953.

95. Stewart, M. J., and Milford, L. W.: Fracture-dislocation of the hip; an end result of study. *J Bone Joint Surg (Am)* 36: 315, 1954.

96. Stewart, W. J. Aseptic necrosis of the head of the femur following traumatic dislocation of the hip joint; Case report and experimental studies. *J Bone Joint Surg* 15: 413, 1933.

97. Stimson, B. B. *Manual of Fractures and Dislocations*, p. 167. Lea & Febiger, Philadelphia, 1939.

98. Stuck, W. G., and Vaughn, W. M. Prevention of disability after traumatic dislocation of the hip. *S Surg* 15: 659–675, 1949.

99. Telfer, N., and Meyers, M. Avascular necrosis and degenerative joint disease. Presented at Northern and Southern California Society of Nuclear Medicine, San Francisco, 1974.

100. Thompson, V. P., and Epstein, H. C. Traumatic dislocation of the hip; a survey of 204 cases covering a period of 21 years. *J Bone Joint Surg (Am)* 33: 746–778, 1951.

101. Tronzo, R. Surgical approaches to the hip joint; a comprehensive review. *J Continuing Educ Orthop* (November), 17–51, 1978.

102. Trueta, J. *Studies of the Development and Decay of the Human Frame.* Saunders, Philadelphia, 1968.

103. Urist, M. R. Injuries to the hip joint/ traumatic dislocations incurred chiefly in Jeep injuries in World War II. *Am J Surg* 74: 586–597, 1947.

104. Urist, M. R. Fractures of the acetabulum; the nature of the traumatic lesion, treatment, and two-year end results. *Am J Surg* 127: 1150–1164, 1948.

105. Urist, M. R. Fracture-dislocation of the hip joint; the nature of the traumatic lesion, treatment, late complications and end results. *J Bone Joint Surg (Am)* 30: 699–727, 1948.

106. Wadsworth, T. G. Traumatic dislocation of the hip with fracture of the shaft of the ipsilateral femur. *J Bone Joint Surg (Br)* 43: 47–49, 1961.

107. Walker, W. A. Traumatic dislocation of the hip joint. *Am J Surg* 50: 545–549, 1940.

108. Watson-Jones, R. *Fractures and Other Bone and Joint Injuries*, ed. 2, p. 619. Williams & Wilkins, Baltimore, 1943.

109. Webber, M. M., and Wagner, J. Early diagnosis of avascular necrosis of the femoral head by radio-isotope methods. (Personal communication.)

110. Westterborn, A. Central dislocation of the femoral head treated with mold arthroplasty. *J Bone Joint Surg (Am)* 36: 307, 1954.

111. Wiltberger, B. R., Mitchell, C. L., and Hedrick, D. W. Fracture of the femoral shaft complicated by hip dislocation; a method of treatment. *J Bone Joint Surg (Am)* 30: 225, 1948.

112. Wilson, J. C. Personal communication (Children's Hospital, Los Angeles).

113. Wolcott, W. E. The evolution of the circulation in the developing femoral head and neck. *Surg Gynecol Obstet* 77: 61–68, 1943.

INDEX